Positioning in a Wheelchair

A Guide for Professional Caregivers of the Disabled Adult

Second Edition

Positioning in a Wheelchair

A Guide for Professional Caregivers of the Disabled Adult

Second Edition

Jan K. Mayall, DipPT/OT
Trillium Lodge
Parksville, British Columbia
Canada

Guylaine Desharnais, BSc, OTR
Banfield Pavilion Extended Care Unit
Vancouver Hospital and Health Sciences Centre
Seating Consultant
Vancouver, British Columbia
Canada

SLACK Incorporated, 6900 Grove Road, Thorofare, NJ, 08086-9447

Acquisitions Editor: Amy E. Drummond
Publisher: John H. Bond
Associate Editor: Jennifer J. Dyer

Mayall, Jan K.
   Positioning in a wheelchair: a guide for caregivers of the disabled adult/by Jan K. Mayall, Guylaine
     Desharnais.—2nd ed.
   p. cm.
   Includes bibliographical references and index.
   ISBN 1-55642-251-2
   1. Wheelchairs. 2. Patients—Positioning. 3. Sitting position. 4. Physically handicapped—Care.
     I. Desharnais, Guylaine. II. Title.
   [DNLM: 1. Posture. 2. Wheelchairs. WE 103 M467p 1994]
RD757.W4M38 1994
617'.0—dc20
DNLM/DLC
for Library of Congress

94-27090
CIP

Printed in the United States of America

Published by: SLACK Incorporated
               6900 Grove Road
               Thorofare, NJ 08086-9447 USA
               Telephone: 856-848-1000
               Fax: 856-853-5991
               World Wide Web: http://www.slackinc.com

   Last digit is print number: 10 9 8 7 6 5 4 3 2

Dedication

To my mother, June, for her encouragement and support.

To my mother, Graziella, avec tout mon amour.

Contents

About the Authors

Guylaine and Jan are occupational therapists who have worked a combined total of 24 years positioning older disabled adults in wheelchairs. They have been guest speakers on positioning for various health care professionals and have given workshops locally and internationally for other therapists. Both have attended many seating symposiums and seating workshops. Recognizing the profound effect of positioning on function and comfort and the lack of available literature on the subject, they decided to share their expertise in this manual.

Acknowledgments

The authors wish to acknowledge with sincere gratitude Hughes Bernier for the drawings, Gaetan Laurendeau and Andrew Neale for the photography, Hazel Broadley for her assistance with editing this manuscript, and the residents of Banfield Pavilion, Vancouver Hospital and Health Sciences Centre, for their patience as we learned and grew together.

Introduction

Many disabled adults sit for hours each day slumped over in wheelchairs that are designed primarily for transportation. Prolonged periods of sitting in such wheelchairs may not only be uncomfortable but could pose multiple health hazards.

Positioning is a major concern to the therapist working with clients in long-term care settings. In many facilities, staff resources, materials, and funding are limited and positioning of the client in the wheelchair is not a priority. With increased attention to the position of the client, many costly interventions may be avoided and the maintenance of independence and quality of life will be optimal.

The purpose of this manual is to enable the therapist to identify a positioning problem, to do a thorough assessment of the client to determine the cause of the problem, and to assess available appliances and techniques to determine the most effective solution. It is intended to assist with clients who have mild to moderate positioning problems. Severely impaired clients may require the services of a specialized seating clinic for a customized insert. Primarily intended for use in long-term care settings, this information will also be useful for therapists in other types of settings or in the community.

In using this manual, it may be tempting to turn directly to the possible solutions in order to deal with a specific problem. Unless the root of the problem is discovered, unnecessary adaptations may be used which may appear to solve the problem on a temporary basis. For example, if the head droops forward, a quick glance might suggest a type of crown head support. With further investigation, it may become apparent that providing stability to the pelvis and positioning of the trunk would alleviate the problem. The reader is advised to make as thorough an assessment as possible to fully understand the basis of the problem. Using a systematic approach to positioning should then provide a clear understanding of how to proceed.

When the ability to experience the world from a standing position is limited, providing a seated environment that can enhance the ability to lead a vibrant, active life is a rewarding challenge.

Objectives

This manual is intended to assure optimal quality of life for the disabled adult by meeting the following objectives:

- Maximizing participation and independence in performing activities of daily living
- Promoting the ability to interact with the environment
- Preventing pressure sores and alleviating pain
- Preventing deformities
- Providing comfort
- Facilitating transfers and mobility
- Assuring safety

Ideally, a client would be positioned to meet all of the above objectives. However, such a situation is seldom the case due to factors such as nonacceptance of a device by the client or limited financial resources. The role of the therapist is to ensure that all potential problems are addressed. To accomplish this, it is essential for the therapist to develop expertise in:

- Performing a thorough assessment of the client
- Analyzing the results of the assessment to determine the cause(s) of the problem(s)
- Assessing the effectiveness and the limitations of available equipment, wheel-chairs, and techniques

This is an ongoing process as the client's status may change and new products constantly appear on the market.

1 | The Importance of Positioning

Sitting is a dynamic, not a static, behavior. When seated, many different postures are assumed and vary according to the activity performed. For example, when sitting at a table engaged in an activity, the upper body is leaning forward with the hips and knees in flexion. When sitting on a chesterfield, the hips and knees are in greater extension. The least amount of energy should be expended in assuming and maintaining the sitting position in order to conserve the maximum amount of energy for other activities. We move a lot when we sit. A disabled person may sit for 3 to 10 hours a day without the ability to reposition himself or herself. Long-term sitting for an able person is usually 1 or 2 hours with shifts in position during that time. Being in a poor posture for a short time is usually not a problem but for longer periods skin, joints, and muscles may become very stressed. The worse the position, the greater the reaction.

Normal postural control enables us:
- To establish a preferred position and a stable base
- To move within that stable base to interact with the environment
- To move between stable positions
- All with minimum energy expenditure

Some of the resulting complications of poor posture are:
- Contractures and deformities
- Tissue breakdown
- Masked ability
- Reduced performance and tolerance
- Infection, urinary tract infection, respiratory insufficiency
- Fatigue and discomfort

These complications may lead to a compromised quality of life, increased cost of care, and an increased care load. The following are examples of how function is affected by positioning:

- When the head droops forward onto the chest, eating becomes difficult and the ability to interact actively and meaningfully with the environment decreases.
- Mobilizing the wheelchair will be very difficult if one foot constantly falls off the footrest and drags on the floor.
- Use of the hands and arms will be affected if the client has a weak trunk and leans to one side.

Therefore, "... good posture positively correlates not only with the integrity of joints, but also with the abilities to experience emotion appropriately, display sound perceptual ability, and experience healthy organic functioning. Since posture has been demonstrated to be a variable in both mental and physical health, the maintenance of good posture should be a priority concern in institutions."[1]

Encouraging the disabled adult to be up out of bed daily will lessen the hazards of immobility (Figure 1-1). The ability to shift position in the wheelchair is a safeguard against the possibility of pressure sores, contractures, loss of sensation, muscle atrophy, and other potential problems. These factors must be taken into consideration when positioning a client. The caregivers must be even more alert when there is lack of independent mobility.

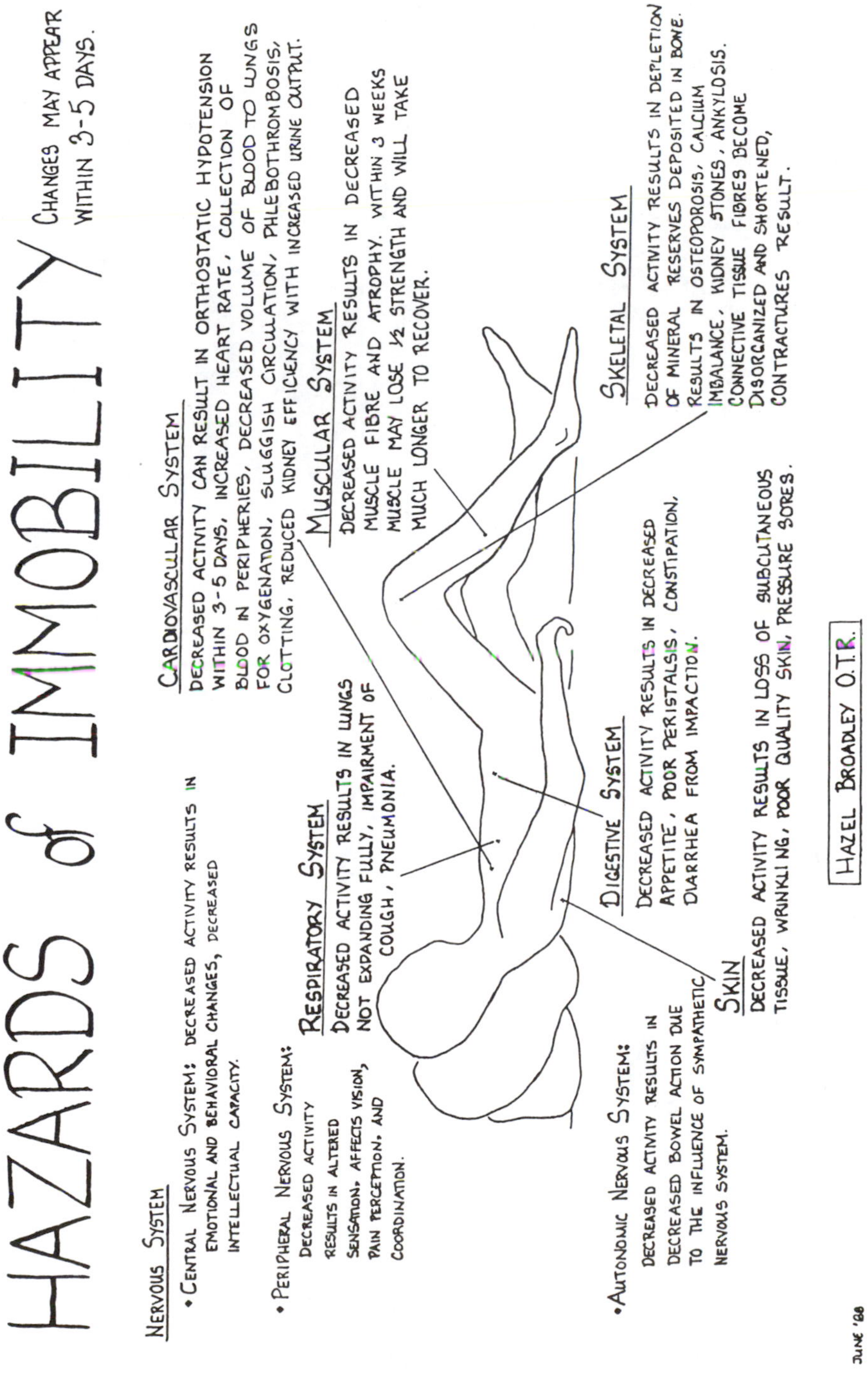

HAZARDS of IMMOBILITY

CHANGES MAY APPEAR WITHIN 3-5 DAYS.

NERVOUS SYSTEM

- CENTRAL NERVOUS SYSTEM: DECREASED ACTIVITY RESULTS IN EMOTIONAL AND BEHAVIORAL CHANGES, DECREASED INTELLECTUAL CAPACITY.

- PERIPHERAL NERVOUS SYSTEM: DECREASED ACTIVITY RESULTS IN ALTERED SENSATION. AFFECTS VISION, PAIN PERCEPTION, AND COORDINATION.

- AUTONOMIC NERVOUS SYSTEM: DECREASED ACTIVITY RESULTS IN DECREASED BOWEL ACTION DUE TO THE INFLUENCE OF SYMPATHETIC NERVOUS SYSTEM.

CARDIOVASCULAR SYSTEM

DECREASED ACTIVITY CAN RESULT IN ORTHOSTATIC HYPOTENSION WITHIN 3-5 DAYS, INCREASED HEART RATE, COLLECTION OF BLOOD IN PERIPHERIES, DECREASED VOLUME OF BLOOD TO LUNGS FOR OXYGENATION, SLUGGISH CIRCULATION, PHLEBOTHROMBOSIS, CLOTTING, REDUCED KIDNEY EFFICENCY WITH INCREASED URINE OUTPUT.

MUSCULAR SYSTEM

DECREASED ACTIVITY RESULTS IN DECREASED MUSCLE FIBRE AND ATROPHY. WITHIN 3 WEEKS MUSCLE MAY LOSE ½ STRENGTH AND WILL TAKE MUCH LONGER TO RECOVER.

SKELETAL SYSTEM

DECREASED ACTIVITY RESULTS IN DEPLETION OF MINERAL RESERVES DEPOSITED IN BONE. RESULTS IN OSTEOPOROSIS, CALCIUM IMBALANCE, KIDNEY STONES, ANKYLOSIS. CONNECTIVE TISSUE FIBRES BECOME DISORGANIZED AND SHORTENED, CONTRACTURES RESULT.

RESPIRATORY SYSTEM

DECREASED ACTIVITY RESULTS IN LUNGS NOT EXPANDING FULLY, IMPAIRMENT OF COUGH, PNEUMONIA.

DIGESTIVE SYSTEM

DECREASED ACTIVITY RESULTS IN DECREASED APPETITE, POOR PERISTALSIS, CONSTIPATION, DIARRHEA FROM IMPACTION.

SKIN

DECREASED ACTIVITY RESULTS IN LOSS OF SUBCUTANEOUS TISSUE, WRINKLING, POOR QUALITY SKIN, PRESSURE SORES.

HAZEL BROADLEY O.T.R.

JUNE '88

Figure 1-1. Hazards of Immobility.

2 Basic Sitting Position in a Wheelchair

An understanding of the basic seated position and the systematic approach are prerequisites to assessing and positioning the disabled client. The systematic approach to positioning is a result of the analysis of the seated posture, the key being the pelvis. This systematic approach provides the framework for the whole process of positioning in a wheelchair. It begins with the pelvis, followed by the lower extremities from proximal to distal, the lower trunk, the upper trunk, the head and neck, and lastly, the upper extremities from proximal to distal.

Following is a description of the normal sitting posture starting with the pelvis, how this applies to wheelchair positioning, and how to measure a client for a wheelchair.

Pelvis

The pelvis provides a stable base, the position of which forms the foundation for the support of the rest of the body. In the normal sitting posture, the pelvis is centered, level in the lateral plane with a slight anterior tilt. The action of sitting causes the pelvis to rotate backward due to the tension in the hamstrings, the posterior thigh muscles. This in turn promotes flexion or flattening of the lumbar spine. Because the hamstrings span the hip and the knee, the degree of hip flexion and knee extension are critical in avoiding overstretching of the hamstrings. A maximum of 100 degrees of hip flexion and 105 degrees of knee extension is advised.

Positioning and Measurement

The hips are positioned in the middle and as far back on the seat as possible so that the pelvis is centered and level. Check to see that the iliac crests are level and aligned from side to side to ensure that there is no lateral rotation of the pelvis. The pelvis should be in a neutral position, i.e., slightly tilted forward. The seat width must allow a 1.25 cm (0.5 in.) clearance on each side. This helps distribute the weight over the widest possible surface and still allows for support of the trunk and upper extremities. Seat depth should allow a 2.5 cm (1 in.) clearance from the back of the knee to the front of the sling seat. This is to distribute the weight evenly along the buttocks and thighs.

Lower Extremities

The pelvis and thighs provide the stable base for sitting. The thighs are parallel to each other and in a neutral position, i.e., no rotation at the hips. This creates a wide base of support. By providing support through the thighs, pressure is reduced over the ischial tuberosities, thus spreading the weight. Correct positioning of the legs and feet also contributes to stability and prevents sliding forward in the wheelchair. The feet rest flat on the floor or footrests with the ankles at 90 degrees.

Positioning and Measurement

When adjusting the footrest height, the client is sitting on a cushion and wearing a pair of shoes or slippers. To confirm that there is good support, check that the femurs are parallel to the seat, that the full length of the thighs is supported on the cushion, and that the feet are resting flat on the footrests. This will encourage weight distribution from the coccyx-ischium region onto the well-padded thighs. The footrests should have at least a 5 cm (2 in.) clearance from the floor. When the client is well positioned the hips will be at about 100 degrees, the knees at 105 degrees, and the ankles at 90 degrees with the heels resting flat on the footrests (Figure 2-1).

Trunk

When the lower half of the body is well positioned and stabilized, the upper half can then be positioned for interaction with the environment.

Position and alignment of the spine are dependent on the position of the pelvis and the integrity of the lumbar lordosis. A level pelvis ensures equal weight bearing through both ischial tuberosities and promotes upper trunk symmetry. The pelvis is tilted slightly forward to promote a lumbar lordosis which in turn dictates the curves of the thoracic and cervical spines. Good sitting posture ensures the same spinal curves that are present in the erect standing position. These curves are as follows: the lumbar spine (the lower five vertebrae) is convex forward, creating a lumbar lordosis; the thoracic spine (the next twelve vertebrae) is slightly concave forward

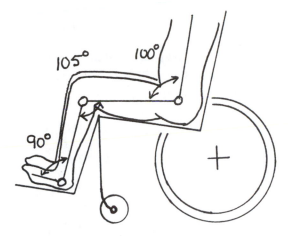

Figure 2-1. Position of lower extremities.

and is called minimal thoracic kyphosis; and the cervical spine (the upper seven vertebrae) is slightly convex forward, creating a minimal cervical lordosis.

Positioning and Measurement

The height of the backrest depends on the amount of trunk support required. The backrest should be as high as necessary for support, as low as possible for function. To check for adequate back support for clients with adequate trunk control, insert the breadth of four fingers (about 10 cm or 4 in.) between the top of the back upholstery to under the axilla.

Head and Neck

The head should be upright and supported by the neck in the midline. The ability to hold the head in the midline is directly dependent on the position of the pelvis, the integrity of the lumbar lordosis and the spine, and the strength of the neck muscles.

Upper Extremities

The manipulative skills of the upper extremities are functionally dependent on the stability and symmetry of the trunk and the ability to control the shoulder girdle to bring the upper extremities and hands into the midline.

For correct armrest height, measure from the seat cushion to just under the elbow, which should be held at a right angle. Add 2.5 cm (1 in.) to that measurement. To confirm the fit, check that with the back resting against the back canvas and forearms supported on the armrests, the shoulder is in approximately 30 degrees flexion and 60 degrees flexion at the elbow. Correct armrest height will help the client maintain good posture and balance. Comfortable support will also be provided to the upper extremities and shoulders.

Ideally, the wheelchair seat should be inclined toward the back by 10 degrees, the legs should be 20 degrees from vertical, and the back 10 to 15 degrees from vertical (Figure 2-2).

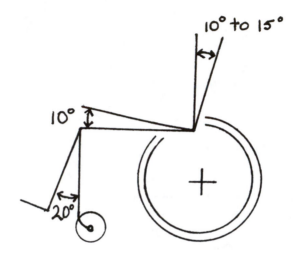

Figure 2-2. Correct wheelchair position.

3 | Types of Wheelchairs

A wheelchair should assure comfort, independence, and maximization of functional abilities. There is a wide variety of wheelchairs on the market and with new technology, materials, research, and increased input from the consumer population, products are constantly changing and improving. Therefore, it is necessary to keep well informed about available products, their advantages and limitations.

A good understanding of the basic seating position combined with a thorough assessment of the client will help determine the most appropriate type of wheelchair. Consideration must be given to the following points when choosing a wheelchair:

- *Portability* Need for the wheelchair to be transported? How heavy is it? How compact is it when folded?
- *Maintenance*. Are parts readily available? Who will do the necessary repairs?
- *Propulsion*. Will it be self-propelled? If so, will the client need special positioning to maintain optimal alignment with the wheels? If propelled by the caregiver, consider the height of the push handles.
- *Size*. Will the wheelchair fit in the client's environment? Door widths? Bathroom? Need for a ramp? Consider the overall width and length of the wheelchair.
- *Trial opportunity*. Is the wheelchair available for a trial period in the client's environment? Trial run through a typical day?
- *Amount*. Would having two or more wheelchairs be a solution for the individual who has a more active lifestyle or varied interests? Consider indoor versus outdoor activity, home versus work versus play environments.
- *Compatibility*. With the advancements in technology, many seated mobility products are intercompatible. The final integrated system can be the result of individually prescribed components.

Following is a short description of several common types of wheelchairs.

Standard Adult Wheelchair

- Regular adult: seat width 46 cm (18 in.), seat height from floor 50 cm (19.75 in.) (Figure 3-1)
- Narrow adult: seat width 41 cm (16 in.), seat height from floor 50 cm (19.75 in.)

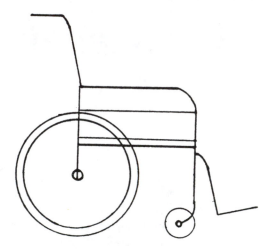

Figure 3-1. Standard adult wheelchair.

Hemi Wheelchair

- Available in regular or narrow adult
- Seat height from floor is 44 cm (17.50 in.), allowing the client to mobilize the wheelchair with one or both lower extremities

Semi-Reclining Wheelchair

- Wheelchair back reclines 30 degrees from vertical and locks in several positions (Figure 3-2)
- Back upholstery is 13 cm (5 in.) higher than a standard adult wheelchair
- Has a detachable 25 cm (10 in.) telescopic headrest
- Rear wheels are set back 3 cm (1.25 in.) to maintain good balance and stability of the wheelchair

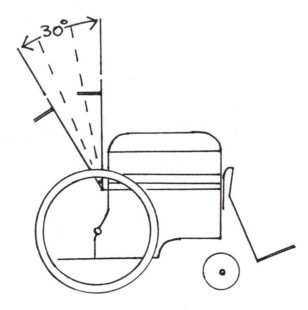

Figure 3-2. Semi-reclining wheelchair.

Fully Reclining Wheelchair

- Wheelchair back reclines to horizontal from vertical position and locks into various positions of recline (Figure 3-3)
- Back upholstery is 17 cm (7 in.) higher than a standard adult wheelchair
- Has a detachable 25 cm (10 in.) telescopic headrest
- Rear wheels are set back 12 cm (5 in.) to maintain stability of the wheelchair

Amputee Wheelchair

- Same width and height as standard adult wheelchair
- Rear wheels set back 3 cm (1.25 in.) to maintain chair stability and to compensate for the loss of the lower extremity(ies) (Figure 3-4)
- If an amputee wheelchair is not available:
    - an amputee adapter (Everest and Jennings) can be fitted to a standard adult wheelchair or
    - add 4.5 to 9 kilos (10 to 20 lbs.) of weight to the footrests

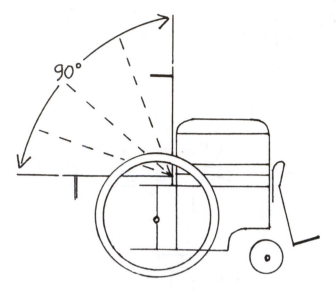

Figure 3-3. Fully reclining wheelchair.

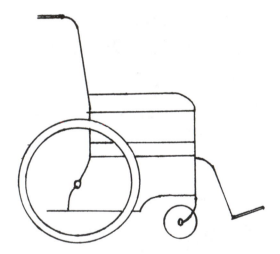

Figure 3-4. Amputee wheelchair.

Lightweight Wheelchair

- Lighter than a standard wheelchair, it is designed for ease of propulsion
- Usually easier to customize as manufacturers offer a wider selection of seat widths and depths, back heights

- Most lightweight wheelchairs come with a fold-up frame
- Often fitted with quick-release wheel-hubs and some horizontal and vertical axle adjustment
- In addition to the usual features of standard wheelchairs, lightweight wheelchairs offer extra options such as a choice of casters, type of foot plates, wheel locks, colors, and type of upholstery. Note that when comparing the weight of various wheelchairs, be aware of whether or not attachments, such as footrests, are included.

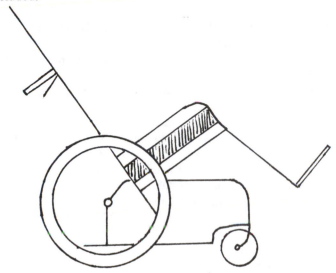

Figure 3-5. Tilt-in-space seating system.

Tilt-in-Space Seating System

The tilt-in-space seating systems (Figure 3-5) are designed to tilt backward without changing or sacrificing the individual's optimal sitting position. The angle between seat, backrest, and leg- or footrest remains the same in all positions.

By increasing the angle of tilt, the weight is redistributed more evenly over a larger surface area, i.e., back, buttocks, and thighs. The blood flow to weightbearing areas, the ischial tuberosities, coccyx, and sacrum, is therefore increased, reducing the risk of a pressure sore. The effect of gravity on the spine in an upright sitting position is alleviated, thus requiring less muscle work to maintain the spine, head, and neck in proper alignment, decreasing the pain and increasing the length of time possible to stay up in the wheelchair.

A wheelchair that can be tilted back while maintaining the optimal sitting position provides a resting position and can be used periodically throughout the day. Tilt-in-space seating systems offer a viable option for severely disabled clients who tire quickly and are unable to shift their weight in the wheelchair by offering the possibility of various and frequent changes of position.

A tilted back position should be used as a resting position only. It does not promote upright and forward sitting which is necessary when participating in table activities, for example. But with a combination of positions, the ability to maintain an upright sitting posture could be increased allowing individuals to improve their level of participation in activities such as meal management.

Tilt-in-space seating systems can be described as follows:
- Various styles of tilting mechanisms:
    - Tilt by pivoting around the seat and back junction
    - The seat and back junction remains level in the horizontal plane and moves forward as the unit tilts backward
    - The seat and back junction is lowered into the frame as the unit tilts
    - The front of the seat does not raise up
- Depending on the tilt-in-space seating system, the amount of tilt ranges from 0 degrees to 30 and 45 degrees.
- Tilt-in-space seating systems wheelbases are either self-propelled, attendant controlled, or mounted on a powered chair base.
- Tilt-in-space mechanisms mounted on a manual chair base are usually attendant operated; they are usually client operated when mounted on a powered chair base.
- Most tilt-in-space seating systems allow for extensive standard customization including varying seat width and depth, back height, footrests or elevating legrests, removable and adjustable headrest, and adjustable height armrests.
- Some seating systems offer a variety of components to choose from and to assemble into a customized system, e.g., the adult MOSS II (Modular Orthotic Seating System II) from Otto Bock (Figure 3-6).
- Some seating systems offer a basic base that can be interfaced with custom or off-the-shelf seating equipment.
- Transportation can be a limiting factor. Some tilt-in-space seating systems cannot be dismantled for transportation or are dismantled in several bulky pieces.

High Performance Wheelchair

High performance wheelchairs (Figure 3-7), often called sports chairs, were designed to improve and enhance mobility primarily with the active younger individual. Now the benefits of using a high performance wheelchair or a wheelchair with similar characteristics are becoming more evident for maximizing independent wheelchair mobility for active individuals of all age groups.

The three main advantages of high performance wheelchairs are lightness of weight, easy maneuverability, and directional stability.

Lightweight
High performance wheelchairs and their various components are made of materials such as aluminum, high grade steel, titanium, and carbon fiber. The main goal is to keep the overall weight to a minimum without sacrificing strength and durability. Less energy is required to accelerate and decelerate when mobilizing the wheelchair. The wheelchair is also lighter to lift in and out of a transporting vehicle.

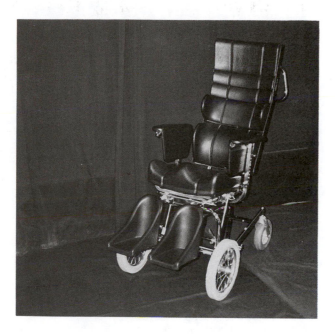

Figure 3-6. Otto Bock adult MOSS II.

Maneuverability

The axle of the rear wheel is moved forward to the back post of the wheelchair. The client's center of gravity is then more in line with the axle line of the wheelchair. This increases the percentage of body weight over the rear wheels and decreases the body weight over the front casters. This shift of body weight to the rear wheels decreases the rolling resistance of the front casters making the wheelchair easier to push.

With the rear wheels more in line with the client's center of gravity, the shoulder joint is directly above the center of the rear wheels allowing for an easier and longer pushing stroke.

Back wheel balance is facilitated with the client's center of gravity more in line with the rear wheels. But some clients may feel uncomfortable as the wheelchair can tip backwards more easily. The further forward the rear wheels are moved, the less the stability.

High performance wheelchairs have a shorter wheelbase. The arm lever required to turn a wheelchair on a shorter base is shorter, thus less effort is required for turning. Also, a short wheelbase requires less space to turn.

The rear wheels have horizontal and vertical axle adjustments. Horizontal axle adjustments are forward adjustments which further decrease the overall length of the

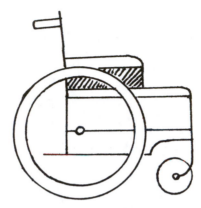

Figure 3-7. High performance wheelchair.

wheelbase and bring the axle line of the wheelchair into closer alignment with the client's center of gravity. Vertical axle adjustment allows the rear wheels to move higher on the frame, lowering the client's center of gravity, thus improving stability. It creates a "bucketing" effect. This can also be achieved by lengthening the front caster forks.

Directional Stability

The rear wheels of a high performance wheelchair are cambered, or angled towards the chair at the top, in order to maximize precise tracking. This is based on the principle that a wheel will run in the direction that it is leaning.

The cambered wheels have the added advantage of being closer to the body. Also, the upper extremities move in the same plane when mobilizing the wheelchair, i.e., extension-abduction of the shoulders to reach the handrims, then push forward, and when the motion is completed the shoulders are in slight flexion-adduction. This allows for a longer and stronger stroke requiring less effort to cover a greater distance.

This completes the basic design of a high performance wheelchair. In addition, the manufacturers offer a wide variety of features and options to allow for custom fitting to better meet the needs of individual clients. But it is of prime importance to remember that there is no best feature or option. The role of the therapist is to help the client choose a wheelchair which best meets his or her needs and lifestyle. Ensure that the client is aware of the possible advantages and disadvantages specific to the type of wheelchair chosen.

The following are points to consider when assessing a client for a high performance wheelchair:

- High performance wheelchairs are generally fitted with quick-release axles on the rear wheels. To maximize strength and rigidity some wheelchairs do not fold. Therefore, if the wheelchair is to be transported, the type of vehicle needs to be determined, how the wheelchair will fit in it, and who is putting the wheelchair in the vehicle.
- Some types of high performance wheelchairs do not offer swinging detachable foot plates which can make standing transfers difficult. They can be fitted with a foot bar or flip-up foot plates and do not allow for unobstructed access to the wheelchair.
- The cambered rear wheels increase the overall width of the wheelchair at the base. This can create spatial difficulties such as going through narrow doorways. Also, the top part of the cambered rear wheels is closer to the seat. This means that anything that overhangs the side of the seat, such as clothing, has a greater chance of rubbing on the wheels.
- When possible, an appropriate wheelchair repair facility should be within the client's vicinity. Parts should be readily available. Note if the client intends to travel within or outside the country of origin.

High performance wheelchairs were primarily designed for active disabled young adults and more often for use in sports. Nowadays, it is becoming widely recognized that all disabled clients who are mobilizing their wheelchairs independently can benefit from using a lighter, custom-fitted wheelchair designed to enhance and optimize mobility. Additionally, one can safely assume that when the wheelchair is easier to maneuver, less energy will be required for mobility and a greater amount of energy will be conserved. This reserve of energy is then available to the client to become more independent and functional within his or her environment and pursue other occupational and leisure activities. In conclusion, a well-chosen and fitted high performance wheelchair can provide the opportunity for greater mobility and improved quality of life.

4 Assessment

Before deciding on the most appropriate positioning intervention, a thorough assessment of the client is necessary to identify his or her seating needs. Secondly, the therapist needs to gain an understanding of the client within his or her environment. The assessment shows how complex the individual is. All facets of the being are dynamic and interrelated. Who is he or she? Where does he or she live? What kinds of places does he or she go to? What does he or she need to do each day? What kinds of equipment does he or she need to use to perform daily activities? The assessment is an interactive process. To prevent fragmentation, ideally, one person who has the necessary skills will follow the client through from the assessment to prescription to follow up. The importance of this relationship cannot be underestimated. To see the client in a whole context in relation to his or her family and community is essential to success. It takes time for relationship building. Put yourself in the mind of the client. Engage that being so you can assist them in realizing their hopes and dreams.

With the information obtained from the assessment, the therapist will:
- Identify the problem and its causes
- Determine the optimal sitting position for the client
- Gain an understanding of the client's needs and potentials for function, present and future

The assessment should include:
- Diagnosis and prognosis
- Age
- Communication status
    preferred language
    verbal and nonverbal expression and comprehension

- Cognitive function
    memory
    learning ability
    problem solving
- Perceptual function
    heminegligence
    body awareness
    apraxia
- Physical ability
    range of motion
    muscle tone
    strength
    pain
    contractures
    sitting tolerance and balance
    standing tolerance and balance
- Level of independence in activities of daily living
- Transfer ability and modality
- Mobility
    ambulation
    wheelchair mobility
- Body weight
- Sensory status
    vision
    hearing
    touch
    (A careful assessment of any area of impaired or absent sensation over the bony prominence such as the ischial tuberosities must be included.)
- Presence of edema in lower and/or upper extremities
- Skin integrity. How often is it checked? By whom? Is there a history of pressure sores? Allergies? Skin graft?
- Leisure interests, lifestyle, indoor/outdoor activities
- Transportation to and from place of residence
- Client's usage of wheelchair. Is the client careless or rough on wheelchair?
- Amount of time spent daily in the wheelchair
- Financial resources of the client

When assessing a client, the therapist should also consider the following points:
- Who initiated the request for the wheelchair positioning assessment? What is perceived as the problem(s) with the present sitting position? Wheelchair? Equipment?
- Consider the reason(s) for the wheelchair positioning assessment. For example, are the abilities changing? Is the need for postural support decreasing or increasing?
- Observe the client's posture in the present seat.
- Examine the wheelchair and the seating without the client. Observing the wheelchair and seating can provide information about its use. Note areas where the

wheelchair and seating is most worn. For example, a pelvic obliquity can be confirmed from the imprint left on a foam cushion.

- Sit the client on a mat table. What is a good sitting position for the client? Keep in mind factors such as normalization of muscle tone, symmetrical sitting posture, and postural control. The goal is to achieve an optimal sitting posture for the client which will:
  - Promote even loading on both sides of the body
  - Maintain alignment of the spine, head, and neck
  - Bring the upper extremities in the midline position

The idea is to restore the body's natural ability to balance itself using minimal adaptation(s).

- Primary caregivers, such as family members and nursing staff, have invaluable information to share since they spend the most time with the client. Consider the role(s) they are going to play in the wheelchair positioning process. What are the physical and psychological capabilities of the caregiver(s) to ensure follow through once the wheelchair positioning is completed.

- The whole process of wheelchair positioning must be client-centered; the client is involved and actively participating in the decision-making process starting with the assessment.

"Cosmesis, an important aspect of seating, is sometimes overlooked by therapists. For example, the choice of covering can be very important even if it is not very important to the provision of seating. The seating system should be considered an extension of the client tastes and self-image. If it meets only the needs of the provider, in terms of usability and appearance, the system will likely be used little."[2]

By allowing time for the understanding of the benefits of proper positioning, the client often will more readily accept the positioning technique or device used.

Following is a wheelchair positioning assessment form used to compile the data collected (Table 4-1).

Based on the data collected and the knowledge of seating and positioning, the therapist will have to customize a solution to suit the client's needs. Because more than one solution can be found suitable for one specific problem, the therapist must have good knowledge of the advantages and disadvantages relevant to each solution. Therefore, we can assume that most solutions to a positioning problem will inevitably include a compromise. Priorities must be clarified. For example, to maximize function, it may be necessary to sacrifice a little spinal alignment or aesthetics. The role of the therapist will be to ensure that while choosing the most appropriate solution, the best compromise will be made. The client and primary caregivers must be aware of the possible disadvantages inherent to any solution adopted. The wheelchair positioning process is depicted in Table 4-2.

TABLE 4-1
WHEELCHAIR POSITIONING ASSESSMENT FORM

Name: _____

Birthdate: _____ Height: _____

Sex: _____ Weight: _____

Address: _____

Postal code: _____ Telephone: _____

Next of kin: _____ Telephone: _____

Referred by: _____ Telephone: _____

Medical history: _____

_____

_____

Preferred language: _____

Communication status: _____

Sensory status:

   Vision: _____

   Hearing: _____

   Touch/pain: _____

Cognitive function:

   Memory: _____

   Learning ability: _____

   Problem solving: _____

Perceptual status:

   Body awareness: _____

   Apraxia: _____

   Perseveration: _____

   Negligence: _____

Transfers: _____

Mobility:

   Ambulation: _____

   Wheelchair: _____

Sitting balance: _____

Time spent in wheelchair daily: _____

Skin integrity: _____

Continence: _____

Living situation (house or apartment, accessibility to or in): _____

_____

_____

Occupational and leisure interests (indoor/outdoor): _____

_____

_____

Transportation (own car): _____

Financial resources: _____

Reason for attending the wheelchair clinic: _____

_____

Wheelchair/equipment tried, used previously: _____

_____

What was good about it? Any problems with it? _____

_____

_____

_____

Power chair: _____

	Problems (Including range of motion, tone, strength, edema, deformity)	Corrective measures
Pelvis		Seat width: _____ depth: _____
Hips		
Knees		
Feet		
Trunk control Spine		Back height: _____
Head/neck		
Shoulder		Armrest height:_____

Arm/hand

_____

Plan: _____

_____

_____

_____

Signature: _____

Date: _____

TABLE 4-2
WHEELCHAIR POSITIONING PROCESS

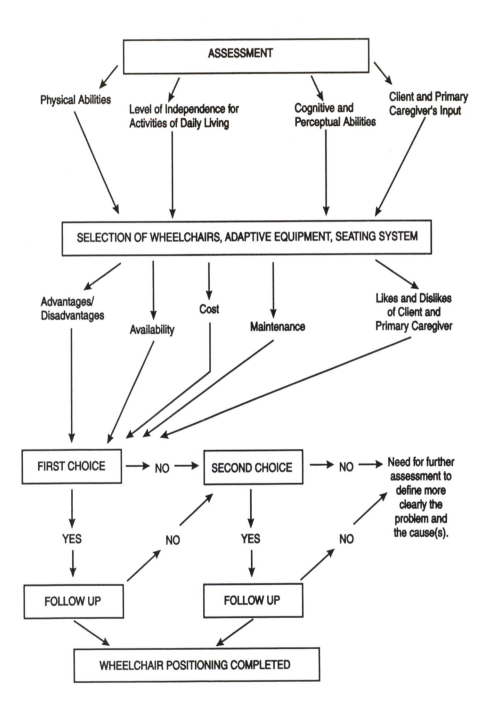

5 Approach to Positioning: Seating the Client

Since the theory and practice of seating and positioning are based on a systematic approach, the following chapters are presented in the same order: pelvis, lower extremities, trunk, head and neck, and upper extremities. Potential problems, special considerations, and possible solutions are discussed for each area.

For each area of difficulty various solutions are described with general recommendations for their possible use. The proposed solutions may serve as a guide to help create new answers to positioning problems and to assist the therapist in analyzing and understanding new wheelchairs, positioning devices, and cushions. Since new products are always coming on the market and available products are being changed and improved, this manual does not contain a complete list of what is presently available. With the understanding gleaned from a thorough assessment of the client, the therapist will be able to assess new equipment to see if it will meet the needs of the client. Most dealers are very helpful regarding specific use of a product, sizes, and changes, and often are able to provide literature about equipment.

Every client is unique and individual, as is every positioning problem. There is no "correct" solution to a specific problem. Keeping in mind that the least amount of intervention is preferable, assess the impact of the adaptation. Is it really necessary? For example, if the pelvis is well supported, another piece of equipment, such as a positioning belt, may become unnecessary. The intention is to facilitate the body's natural ability to maintain the upright position.

Positioning devices are used to enhance function or to provide safety, e.g., to prevent pressure sores and contractures. However, adaptive equipment that limits a client's active movement must be monitored continuously. If, for example, head control is inconsistent and immobilization of the head deemed necessary for meal management, after the meal the device may need to be removed to encourage active head control. Also, the client's condition may improve, thus no longer requiring the use of such a device.

Before selecting a positioning device, e.g., a cushion, it is necessary for the therapist to assess the possible solutions in terms of advantages and disadvantages, possibilities and limitations, and potential clinical applications. Consider the following factors:

- Cost
- Availability
- Maintenance, adjustments. Who is responsible for the upkeep?
- Client and primary caregiver preferences
- Client's level of functioning versus the specific advantages and disadvantages of a possible solution
- The possibility of a trial period

Since no solution will be without disadvantages, it is the therapist's responsibility to carefully assess and communicate the pros and cons of a solution with the client and primary caregiver(s) so they are fully aware of all the implications of the decision.

Pelvis

The pelvis is the foundation on which the trunk is balanced, thus pelvic positioning and stability are prerequisites to performing functional activities involving the upper extremities and/or head. But when assuming an upright sitting posture, the sitting base, i.e., the pelvis and thighs, will carry a large amount of the individual body weight, i.e., trunk, head, and upper extremities, which is situated from and above the pelvis. The pelvic structure contains bony prominences which are or can become weight-bearing areas. These bony prominences, e.g., ischial tuberosities, cannot sustain high and continuous pressure without consequently damaging the surrounding tissue. Therefore, the function of a wheelchair cushion is to provide positioning and stability to the sitting base and pressure relief to the bony prominences of the pelvis. It is then reasonable to say that a wheelchair should not be prescribed without a cushion.

When deciding on the most appropriate type of cushion for a client, a thorough assessment is essential as the solution to a specific problem(s) will vary according to its cause(s) and choices will be influenced by the individual's needs and lifestyle.

Positioning the Pelvis

Because the pelvis is the base, the position of which dictates the position and alignment of body segments, special consideration is given to better understand its functioning. The following is a short explanation of some biomechanical principles on positioning, supporting, and stabilizing the pelvis.

When sitting, the pelvis rests on the ischial tuberosities which can be compared to small rockers. The pelvis is stabilized in a slight anterior tilt by muscle activity, the position of the femurs, and a firm seat and back support.

The main muscle groups which mobilize and stabilize the pelvis are as follows:
- Anterior pelvic tilt
    - Rectus femoris, one of the quadriceps, is a two-joint muscle. Action: flexion of the hip, extension of the knee.
    - Iliopsoas. Action: flexion of the hip.
- Posterior pelvic tilt
    - Gluteus maximus. Action: extension of the hip.
    - Hamstrings are a two-joint muscle. Action: extension of the hip, flexion of the knee.

Depending on the current status of the neuromusculoskeletal system, the ability to stabilize the pelvis in a slightly tilted forward position can be compromised. For example, high tone in the extensor muscles of the trunk and the hips or hamstrings, which pull the pelvis into a posterior tilt, are often encountered.

Proper positioning of the femurs contributes to pelvic stability. They must be parallel to the seat to help balance the pelvis on the ischial tuberosities (Figure 5-1).

When sitting on a level cushion, the femurs slope downward, resulting in increased hip extension. This can be explained as follows (Figure 5-2): the distance from the hip joint to the ischial tuberosities is greater than the distance from the femur or thigh proximal to the knee joint to the top of the cushion. The femurs are therefore unable to participate in stabilizing the pelvis. Stability is then mainly provided by muscle activity which is compromised in the disabled adult. Also, impaired muscle activity patterns can be stimulated, e.g., high tone in the hamstrings.

If the height of the footrest is increased to bring the femurs parallel to the cushion, less weight is taken by the thighs and more weight is taken through the ischial tuberosities. To alleviate this situation, a pre-ischial bar can be used to keep the

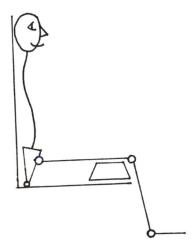

Figure 5-1. Pelvis positioning with a pre-ischial bar.

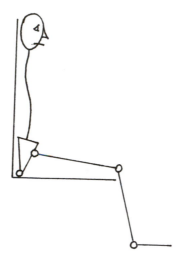

Figure 5-2. Pelvis positioning without a pre-ischial bar.

femurs parallel to the seat. This takes some of the weight off the sacral, coccygeal, and ischial area and moves it forward to be supported by the well-padded thighs (see Figure 5-1). This is referred to as weight redistribution or loading of the thighs.

With the use of a pre-ischial bar, the femurs can assist in stabilizing the pelvis. In turn, the pelvis will rely less on muscle activity for stability and often the occurrence of impaired muscle activity patterns are reduced as the client feels secure, comfortable, and stable sitting in the wheelchair. Several cushions incorporate a pre-ischial bar and are often referred to as positioning cushions. They include: foam cushion with pre-ischial bar, ramp, KSS seat base, the Jay cushions, and the Bard flotation cushion.

Consideration must be given to the following factors when choosing a cushion with a pre-ischial bar:

- Standing transfers can be more difficult because of the 'bucket effect' created by the pre-ischial bar.
- Height of the knees is increased and can create environmental difficulties such as getting close to a table.
- Use of the pre-ischial bar can impede wheelchair mobility with the lower extremities.

The sling seat and back of the wheelchair promote a posterior pelvic tilt thus decreasing the lumbar lordosis, promoting a kyphotic posture, and encouraging sliding forward and out of the wheelchair.

As the back canvas stretches, the pelvis is pulled into a posterior pelvic tilt. Concurrently, the sling seat brings the thighs into adduction with increased hip extension as evidenced by the femurs sloping downward (Figure 5-3).

The use of a contoured firm seat base and back support assist in positioning the pelvis in a slight anterior tilt, in maintaining the femurs parallel to the seat, and in minimizing the muscle activity necessary to stabilize the pelvis (Figure 5-4).

It is preferable to use contoured seats and backs. This increases the surface contact

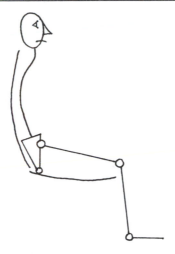

Figure 5-3. Pelvis positioning with sling seat and back.

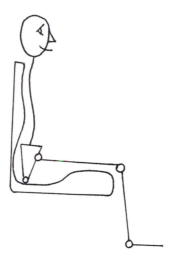

Figure 5-4. Pelvis positioning with contoured firm seat and back.

with the body thereby increasing comfort and decreasing the risk of skin breakdown especially over spinal prominences, ischials tuberosities, coccyx, and sacrum. For contoured firm back support, see page 86 (Trunk, Possible Solutions). For contoured firm seat base, see page 37 (Pelvis, Possible Solutions).

Potential Problems

Pressure Sores

Pressure sores or decubitus ulcers "are localized areas of cellular necrosis almost always occurring over bony prominences."[3]

The two main factors that contribute to pressure sore formation are continuous direct pressure and shearing forces. Problems related to pressure on the tissue vary in degree from redness of the skin on the buttocks to pressure sores and skin breakdown that results in decreased sitting tolerance.

The parts of the body at risk for pressure sores are the areas over the ischial tuberosities, coccyx, sacrum, and the trochanters. Common causes of pressure sores in wheelchairs include:

- Immobility. Inability to shift weight.
- Minimal adipose tissue and/or loss of muscle mass over the buttocks.
- Pelvic obliquity (Figure 5-5) which is caused by the "hammock effect" of the sling seat. It results in increased pressure over one ischial tuberosity and trochanter. This is often accompanied by sideways shearing forces.
- Pressure sores over the sacrum may be caused by a slumped sitting posture or sacral sitting. The shearing forces created by the posterior pelvic tilt as the client tends to slide out of the wheelchair also contribute to the formation of a sacral pressure sore.
- Poor health status.

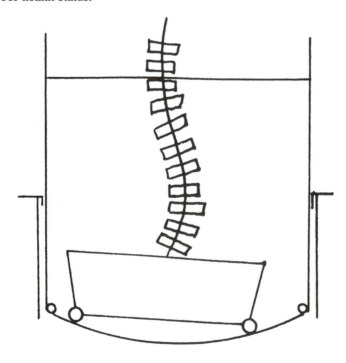

Figure 5-5. Pelvic obliquity.

Poor Sitting Posture

The Hammock Effect

The hammock effect of the wheelchair's sling seat is the primary cause of poor sitting posture. The pelvis may tilt to one side, pelvic obliquity, causing the upper body to lean to the side with an accompanying increased lateral curvature of the spine or scoliosis. The hammock effect also encourages hip adduction and internal rotation. Sitting balance will be affected due to the decreased base of support. The hammock effect also encourages sacral sitting, posterior pelvic tilt, and a rounding out of the lower spine or flattening of the lumbar lordosis which may become a source of discomfort.

Sacral Sitting—The Slider

The slider slips forward in the wheelchair often ending up with the buttocks on the front of the seat, the weight on the sacrum, the feet out on the floor in front or behind the footrests, and the shoulders halfway down the back of the wheelchair. It is a positioning problem very often encountered in long-term care facilities and therefore needs greater attention. Various factors can cause a client to slide in the wheelchair.

- Hypertonicity of the extensor muscles of the hips or extension contractures of the hips limit the ability to attain the sitting position. Compensating for the lack of flexion at the hips, the pelvis is tilted backward increasing flexion of the lumbar spine.
- Inability to extend the knee beyond 90 degrees. Limited knee extension is often due to hypertonicity or shortening of the hamstrings (two-joint muscles), resulting in posterior pelvic tilt, increased hip extension, and knee flexion. It can be accompanied by knee flexion and hip extension contractures. Clients may experience discomfort when they try to extend their knees to enable their feet to rest flat on the foot plates. They will slide forward in the wheelchair to increase knee flexion and to release the tension.
- With hypotonicity or weakness of the trunk and muscles of the lower extremities the client may be unable to stop sliding down in the wheelchair.
- Occasionally a client may slide down in the wheelchair in order to get attention.
- Medical problems that may be contributing to discomfort in the sitting position should be considered. Some clients may have difficulty communicating exactly why they are restless. For example, a client with back pain may slide forward to ease the pain but may be unable to push back up in the wheelchair.
- The client may slide forward in the wheelchair when attempting to mobilize the wheelchair with the lower extremities. To provide freedom of movement for the lower extremities, the buttocks will be moved forward in the wheelchair.

"Wind Swept" Deformity

This is marked by one hip abducted and one hip adducted causing the legs to appear unequal in length. This complex problem is evidenced by:

- Pelvic obliquity and rotation. Check the alignment of the anterior superior iliac spines.
- Poor trunk alignment accompanied by discomfort.
- Increased risk of pressure sores over one ischial tuberosity.

Factors contributing to the wind swept deformity:
- Muscle imbalance due to cerebrovascular accident or multiple sclerosis, for example.
- Spinal deformity such as scoliosis.
- Short wheelchair seat depth which often occurs with clients who are tall or have excessive adipose tissue on the buttocks.
- Mobilizing the wheelchair with one lower extremity, the other lower extremity remaining on the footrest.

The potential problems described above lead to one main problem for the client: poor sitting posture in the wheelchair causing discomfort and limited sitting tolerance.

Special Considerations

- When choosing a cushion, consideration should be given to the following factors:
  - Whether the client is continent
  - How easily the cushion can be cleaned
  - Whether the cushion requires maintenance
  - The weight of the cushion (if it is necessary to transfer the cushion)
  - Cost
  - Durability
- A cushion should not be overlayered because this will cause it to lose its property of pressure relief.
- When cushion covers are necessary, two-way stretch material should be used to prevent shearing forces in any direction and to allow conformity with minimal increase in pressure. Consider the type of two-way stretch material used. For example, nylon reduces friction and facilitates movement in the wheelchair but it may also facilitate sliding.
- It is advisable to secure the cushion to the wheelchair. Since the cushion can slide forward or backward with the client, all four corners require fastening.
- To stabilize the client in the wheelchair, the feet must be comfortably positioned and resting flat on the footrests. By changing the cushion or the base of support the height of the seat may alter and therefore the height of the footrests will require adjustment. When footrests are too high the thighs do not support sufficient body weight, thus increasing the pressure on the ischial tuberosities. If the footrests are too low the feet do not support body weight and the pressure is increased under the thighs. It becomes difficult for the client to push back and sit upright in the wheelchair as well, thus encouraging sliding forward.
- Is the seat depth correct? If the seat is too short the thighs will not be fully supported increasing the pressure under the buttocks as the sitting surface is decreased. If the seat is too long the front edge of the seat canvas will press against the back of the knee causing discomfort and encouraging sliding forward and out of the wheelchair.
- When determining the appropriate length of a wheelchair cushion, the therapist may consider making the cushion 2.5 to 5 cm (1 to 2 in.) longer than the wheelchair seat depth. This will have the following effects:

- Increasing the seat depth to accommodate the thigh length of taller clients.
- Providing postural stability by maintaining an optimal seating surface.

Often, as a client transfers into a wheelchair, the seat cushion slides back by 2.5 to 5 cm (1 to 2 in.) in the space created by the sling back thus decreasing the seating surface by a similar amount under the thighs. This in turn increases pressure under the buttocks and may cause postural instability. Making a cushion longer than the seat canvas can only be accomplished with firm cushions such as a 7.5 cm (3 in.) foam cushion or a Jay cushion. It cannot be done with a soft and pliable cushion such as the Roho dry flotation cushion.

- Positioning belt. Exercise caution when using restraints in a wheelchair as a positioning device for the pelvis. Some clients may become restless and fight against the restraint possibly encouraging what you are trying to prevent, e.g., sliding forward in the wheelchair. Any restraint will interfere with the client's freedom of movement. Careful thought and assessment are necessary when considering this alternative.

- Before ordering, cushions should be tested to ensure that pressure relief and stability are provided.

Possible Solutions

- Cushions
    - Polymer foam
    - Ramp cushion
    - Foam cushion with pre-ischial bar
    - Wedge foam cushion
    - KSS seat base (Special Health Systems)
    - Roho cushion (Roho Inc)
    - Bard flotation cushion (Maddak)
    - Jay cushions (Jay Medical Ltd)
    - J-2 cushion (Jay Medical Ltd)
    - Jay Care cushion (Jay Medical Ltd)
- Level base of support
    - Plywood board
    - Wedge board with foam cushion
    - Champher foam base
    - QA2 seat base (QA2 Seating System)
    - SHS cushion (Special Health Systems)
- Drop seat base
    - Wooden drop seat
    - QA2 drop seat base (QA2 Seating System)
    - SHS fiberglass low seat (Special Health Systems)
- Jay adjustable solid seat (Jay Medical Ltd)
- Long seat base
- Adjustable suspension hooks
- 45 degree lap belt (Special Health Systems)

Cushions

According to several studies,[4-6] no type of cushion is superior at relieving pressure for all clients. The ideal cushion would distribute pressure evenly over the largest skin area. All cushions available to date have positive and negative features. To determine the most appropriate type of cushion an assessment is necessary to meet individual needs and ensure good posture and pressure relief. The assessment should include:

- Diagnosis
- Number of hours spent in the wheelchair daily
- Bladder and bowel control
- History of skin breakdown
- Body build
- Postural problems
- Climate
- Care and maintenance

The cushions described can be divided into three categories:

- Polymer foam
- Air-filled
- Flotation: filled with gel, water, or other type of fluid

Polymer Foam

Polymer foam cushion is the standard wheelchair cushion. Polymer foam is lightweight, breathable, and inexpensive. It is easily modified to the needs of the individual client by cutting, wedging, or gluing.

Foam cushions are not washable and they wear out faster than other types of cushion. As they are lightweight it may be necessary to tie the cushions to the wheelchair to prevent them from sliding forward or backward. A standard wheelchair cushion is made of 7.5 cm (3 in.) medium density foam.

Ramp Cushion

A ramp cushion or pre-ischial bar is usually used in conjunction with a 7.5 cm (3 in.) foam cushion (Figure 5-6) but can also be used with other cushions such as the Roho dry flotation cushion.

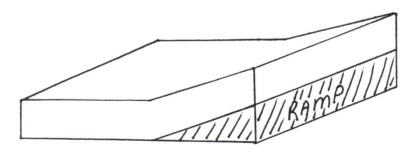

Figure 5-6. Ramp cushion with 7.5 cm foam cushion.

The ramp is placed under the front half of the seat cushion. The posterior half of the cushion remains flat on the seat to facilitate symmetrical horizontal weight bearing through the ischial tuberosities.

The ramp promotes hip flexion which supports the femurs in the horizontal plane. The use of a ramp cushion encourages a better pelvic position, control, and stability. It discourages sacral sitting and sliding forward and out of the wheelchair. The ramp transfers weight from the sacral, coccygeal, and ischial regions to the back of the well-padded thighs.

When using a ramp, standing transfers and mobilizing the wheelchair with the lower extremities may become difficult because of the bucket effect created. Footrest height will need to be readjusted.

Construction:
1. A ramp cushion is made of extra firm chip foam (reconstituted polyether foam).
2. It is cut to the width of the seat cushion. The ramp is 5 cm (2 in.) high at the front tapered down to 0 at the back. The length is on average 20 cm (8 in.) or from 2.5 cm (1 in.) behind the knees to just in front of the gluteal crease.
3. The ramp is covered with a durable fabric and ties are sewn in all four corners to secure it to the wheelchair seat. Alternatively, the ramp can be glued to a seat base, i.e., a board or a champher foam base.

Foam Cushion With Pre-Ischial Bar

The foam cushion with pre-ischial bar (Figure 5-7) is used to counteract forward sliding and the development of redness over the posterior aspect of the buttocks due to mild problems of sacral sitting. The pre-ischial bar transfers the pressure from the sacral, coccygeal, and ischial areas to the back of the well-padded thighs. It maintains the femurs parallel to the seat which in turn will assist in stabilizing the pelvis. A hole is made at the back of the cushion to further decrease the pressure over the sacral and coccygeal region.

The foam cushion with pre-ischial bar can be used with any standard adult wheelchair or reclining wheelchair. After the cushion is fitted, footrest height may need to be adjusted to the increased seat height. The cushion should be attached to the back of the wheelchair frame to prevent it from sliding forward with the client.

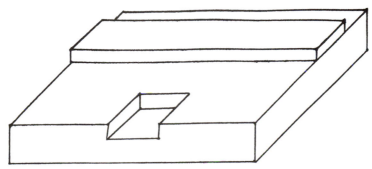

Figure 5-7. Foam cushion with pre-ischial bar.

Construction:
1. A cushion is cut to fit the size of the wheelchair seat out of 7.5 cm (3 in.) medium density foam.
2. A piece of medium density foam 3.5 cm (1.5 in.) high, 12.5 cm (5 in.) wide, and the same width as the cushion is glued 2.5 cm (1 in.) from the front end.
3. A space 5 cm (2 in.) wide, 5 cm (2 in.) long, and 2.5 cm (1 in.) deep is cut in the middle at the back (see Figure 5-7).
4. The cover is made of a durable and stretchable fabric. Ties are sewn in all four corners to attach the cushion to the wheelchair (Figure 5-8).

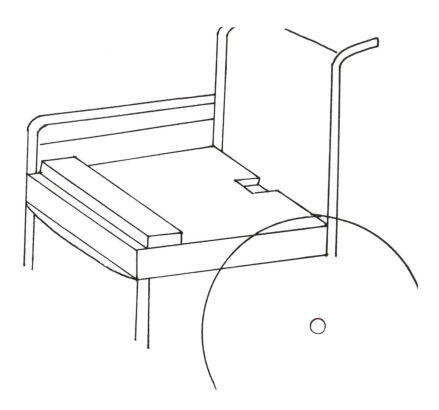

Figure 5-8. Foam cushion with pre-ischial bar.

Wedge Foam Cushion

A wedge foam cushion (Figure 5-9) is a simple solution for mild problems of sacral sitting. It will help to maintain the hips as far back on the seat as possible.

A wedge cushion is more often used with a reclining wheelchair to maintain hip flexion at about 100 degrees.

The cushion should be tied to the back frame of the wheelchair to prevent it from sliding forward with the client. The footrest height should be adjusted to

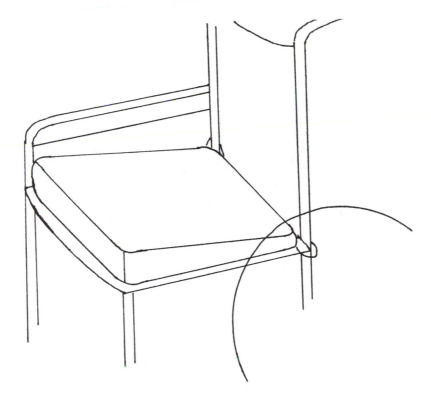

Figure 5-9. Wedge foam cushion.

accommodate the increased seat height caused by the wedge cushion. To avoid increasing the seat height, a drop seat can be fitted.

Construction:

1. A wedge cushion is cut out of medium density foam to fit the size of the wheelchair seat.
2. To maintain 100 degrees of hip flexion the foam is 5 cm (2 in.) thick at the back and 10 to 15 cm (4 to 6 in.) thick at the front depending if using a standard or reclining wheelchair.
3. The cushion is covered with a durable and stretchable fabric. Slippery fabric such as nylon should be avoided.
4. Ties are sewn in all four corners of the cover to secure the cushion to the wheelchair frame.

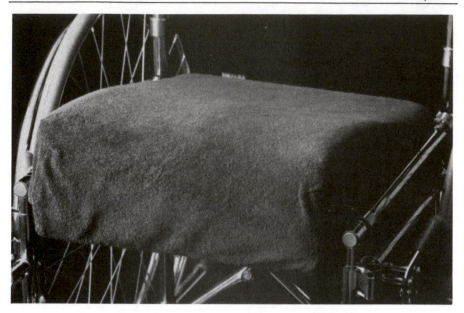

Figure 5-10. KSS seat base.

KSS Seat Base (Special Health Systems)

The KSS seat base (Figure 5-10) is a positioning cushion made of foam on a solid plywood base.

The cushion has an anterior wedge to prevent pelvic tilting or sliding. It also has a firm pre-ischial bar that transfers pressure from the sacral, coccygeal, and ischial region to the back of the well-padded thighs.

The cushion has leg channels to provide a balanced neutral leg position and prevent rotation at the hips.

Assembly:

1. The KSS seat base is made of 5 cm (2 in.) medium density foam and a layer of 2.5 cm (1 in.) comfort foam. The pre-ischial bar is made of 2.5 cm (1 in.) medium density foam.
2. After the sling seat is removed, the KSS seat base is suspended on the wheelchair frame with four stainless steel snap-on suspension hooks.
3. The cushion has a stretch terry cover over a water-resistant neoprene shell. The KSS seat base can be fitted to most types of standard adult or reclining wheelchairs. It is available in two standard sizes: 41 and 46 cm (16 and 18 in.) wide.

Roho Cushion (Roho Inc)

The Roho cushion is a system of soft, flexible, and interconnected air cells designed to distribute the body weight and relieve peak pressure on bony parts of the body. It is not a cushion for sitting "on" but rather a cushion for sitting "in." The immersion assures maximum skin contact and conformity and maintains pelvic stability.

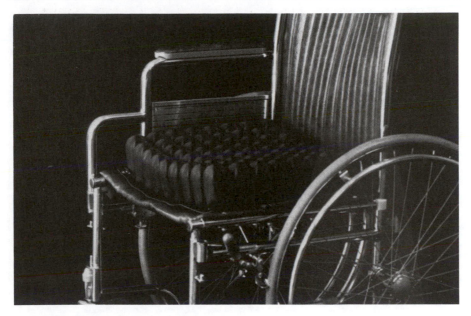

Figure 5-11. High profile Roho cushion.

The Roho cushion does not provide stability and therefore is not recommended for clients who slide forward in their wheelchair or who have a poor sitting position due to increased extensor tone. However, seating instability can be the result of overinflation of the cushion.

Some clients may experience difficulty transferring sideways to another surface as the Roho cushion is a soft and moving surface.

These cushions are lightweight, easy to clean, and easy to transfer. The air pressure needs to be checked regularly to assure correct pressure and to maximize sitting stability.

Roho Inc offers a variety of types and sizes of cushions. Customized cushions are also available to meet the needs of the individual client.

The following is a short description of commonly used Roho cushions:

- The high profile Roho cushion (Figure 5-11) remains the cushion of choice in preventing and healing decubitus ulcers in long-term or high-risk sitting. The cushion is made of 10 cm (4 in.) high air cells.
- The low profile Roho cushion is for active clients with a potential risk of pressure sores. The cushion is made of 5 cm (2 in.) high air cells.
- The high profile or low profile dual manifold cushion is divided into two segments with one valve each that is adjusted individually. It can be used to provide side-to-side or front-to-back control. The cushion is useful in the positioning of the unilateral amputee or the client with scoliosis as it accommodates asymmetry in sitting. It can also be used to prevent sacral sitting and sliding forward in the wheelchair.
- The Roho enhancer cushion (Figure 5-12) is designed to promote good sitting posture. The cushion is made of 5, 7.5, and 10 cm (2, 3, and 4 in.) high cells and

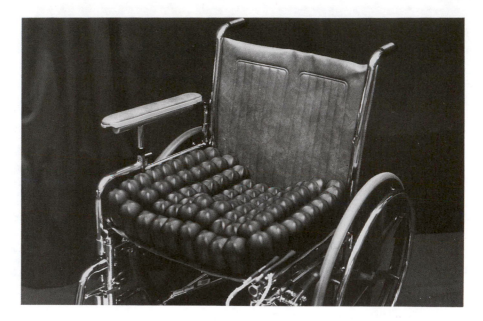

Figure 5-12. Roho enhancer cushion.

two manifolds. One interior manifold adjusts for tissue viability in high-risk areas i.e., coccyx, ischial tuberosities, and perineal areas. The perimeter manifold adjusts for stability and enhanced positioning. The different height cells are positioned to recreate a pre-ischial bar, midline channeling of the legs, and provide lateral and pelvic stability.

- The Roho cover helps protect the cushion surface and keeps the cushion's cells from protruding beyond the wheelchair seat. The top of the cover is made of a two-way stretch fabric and the bottom is made of a non-skid material to prevent the cushion from sliding in the wheelchair. The Roho cushion cover can also be used with other types of cushions such as customized foam.

Assembly:

1. Inflate the cushion until the middle of the cushion begins to arch slightly.
2. Sit the client on the inflated cushion.
3. Insert one hand under the buttocks, palm upward, finger tips touching one ischial tuberosity.
4. The cushion is deflated until the clearance between the bony prominence and the base of the cushion is one finger's thickness (1.2 cm or 0.5 in.).

Bard Flotation Cushion (Maddak)

The Bard flotation cushion (Figure 5-13) is recommended for clients who require stabilization of the pelvis and who are also at risk for pressure sores.

The Bard flotation cushion comes in two parts: a water-filled cushion and an air frame. The water-filled cushion assures even pressure distribution. The air-filled frame helps to prevent sacral sitting and sliding forward in the wheelchair by

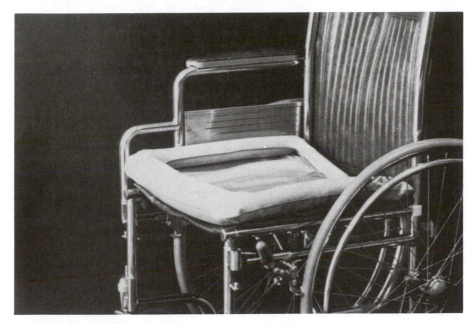

Figure 5-13. Bard flotation cushion.

maintaining the femurs parallel to the seat. It can also be effective in preventing sliding when 100 degrees of hip flexion cannot be achieved due to mild extension contractures. If extension contractures are severe other approaches or adaptations need to be considered.

The Bard flotation cushion does not slide or move in the wheelchair due to its weight and therefore can prevent sliding of clients who have increased extensor tone or extensor spasm in the lower extremities or of the whole body. But, it may be too heavy for clients who need to transfer the cushion independently.

The Bard flotation cushion is available in one standard adult size: 46 x 41 cm (18 x 16 in.). It can be used with any type of adult wheelchair 46 cm (18 in.) wide. When fitting the Bard flotation cushion, the footrest height will need to be adjusted to the increased seat height. It is not advisable to use the Bard flotation cushion with very heavy clients.

Assembly:

Since the cushion is filled with water some clients may find it pleasantly cool while others may find it cold. A sheet of 0.5 cm (3/16 in.) thick low temperature closed-cell foam such as plastazote can be used to insulate the water-filled cushion. To maximize the effectiveness of the cushion the cover used should be of durable and stretchable fabric.

Jay Cushions (Jay Medical Ltd)

Jay cushions are designed to provide postural support and pressure relief for clients at high risk for skin problems from sitting in a wheelchair for prolonged periods.

Jay cushions consist of two parts: a contoured foam base and a flolite pad. Flolite is a fluid within the pad which has no memory thus providing optimal conformation. The flolite pad has a center seam to stop the fluid moving from side to side and to prevent the fluid from moving away from a lean. The flolite is wider than the base allowing it to be pocketed in the rear depression of the foam base. This ensures that the ischial tuberosities and coccyx are totally immersed in the pad with no hammocking or increased surface resistance. The flolite is slow flowing. It moves with the client but stability is not sacrificed.

The contoured foam base has a slight backward angle and a rear depression. The pelvis is positioned lower than the legs, putting the hips into flexion and keeping the femurs parallel to the seat. This helps to stabilize the pelvis, decreasing the risk of sliding forward and out of the wheelchair and providing trunk stability. The foam base has sculptured leg channels which encourage a neutral leg position. Since it is firm, the solid foam base can overhang the sling seat by 5 cm (2 in.) thus allowing the use of a longer cushion to accommodate, for example, the thigh length of taller clients.

The Jay cushion comes with a breathable cover that reduces perspiration and heat build-up. The non-skid bottom prevents the cushion from sliding in the wheelchair. The cushion is easy to clean and needs to be stored flat.

There are two types of Jay cushions: the Jay cushion and the Jay Active cushion. The original Jay cushion (Figure 5-14) is designed to provide optimal seating posture, postural control, and pressure relief. Certain clients may find the cushion heavy when transferring it on and off their wheelchairs. When clients are fitted with "snug" fitting wheelchairs, they may end up sitting on the sloped sides of the contoured base which can cause excessive trochanteric pressure and lead to a pressure sore.

The Jay Active cushion has a lighter and softer foam base with a curved bottom which compensates for the hammock effect of the sling seat. The flolite pad

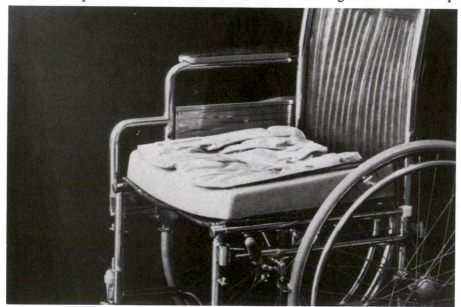

Figure 5-14. Original Jay cushion.

covers only the rear depression of the foam base. The adductor leg wedges are removable to adjust leg position. Some clients may find the Jay Active cushion easier to transfer on and off as it has softer contouring and a narrower profile. However, the Jay Active cushion does not offer the postural support provided by the original Jay cushion.

The Jay recliner cushion is similar to the original Jay cushion except that the flolite pad has an extra segment across the middle of the back of the fluid pad. Also called "quadrant pad," it prevents fluid from bottoming out during reclining by limiting front-to-back movement of the flolite.

The Jay cushions are available in a wide variety of standard sizes from 31.5 to 61 cm (12 to 24 in.) wide and from 28 to 51 cm (11 to 20 in.) deep. Check with a Jay Medical dealer for an up-to-date list of available cushions and sizes.

Assembly:

When assessing for a Jay cushion, sit the client on the cushion without its cover for 2 minutes. Transfer the client out of the wheelchair and look at the flolite pad. At least 0.6 cm (0.25 in.) of fluid should remain where the ischials and coccyx were positioned. Also, check where the ischials and coccyx were positioned on the flolite pad; they should be centered on the posterior part of the pad. The ischials of clients who are sacral sitters tend to hit the central slope of the posterior depression. The cushion can be moved forward in the wheelchair and a foam bar can be added to fill the space left behind the cushion.

Clients who are thin and bony are more inclined to "bottom out" the Jay cushion. Fluid supplement pads can be added to the cushion. Refer to the Jay information material on how to use the supplement pads. Single, double, or triple overfilled pads are available. The single overfilled pad is the most frequently used.

The Jay box contains accessories to customize a cushion to better meet the positioning needs of the individual client. The accessories adhere to the foam base with Velcro. They include a solid seat insert, a wedge base, fluid supplement pads, adductor wedges, an abductor build-up, hip guides, and pelvic obliquity build-ups. It is also possible to custom cut the solid foam base to accommodate, for example, leg length discrepancy. It is necessary to recoat the cut with a special Jay vinyl paint to restore its waterproof property.

Custom sizes and custom cut Jay cushions are available. Ask a Jay Medical dealer about feasibility and for information hand-outs and videos that further explain assessment and fitting of Jay Medical equipment.

J-2 Cushion (Jay Medical Ltd)

Similar to the original Jay cushion, the J-2 cushion (Figure 5-15) is designed to provide postural support and pressure relief for clients at high risk for skin problems from sitting in a wheelchair for prolonged periods of time.

The J-2 cushion consists of two parts: a contoured base and a J-2 fluid pad. This fluid is low maintenance, i.e., does not require regular kneading, and maintains its viscosity at high and low temperatures. The J-2 pad is divided into three sections to better maintain the fluid under the ischial tuberosities and coccygeal area and to eliminate the need for quadrant pads. See page 45 (Pelvis, Jay Cushions) for more information. Inside the pad, there is a soft contoured foam that is located under the

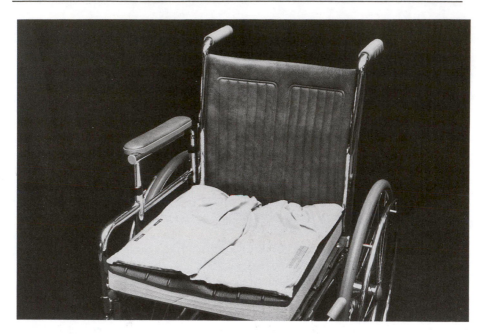

Figure 5-15. J-2 cushion.

thighs and trochanter for extra comfort. This molded foam provides self-adjustment of the cushion minimizing the risk of bottoming out the J-2 fluid pad. The contoured foam is only slightly compressed under a thin person which minimizes the rear well size and helps to concentrate the Jay flow fluid under the buttocks. A heavier person compresses the foam to a greater degree. The resulting increase in well area allows greater immersion into the fluid.

The contoured foam base is made of a light, durable, molded, closed-cell foam. The base has a slight backward angle and a rear depression. The rear depression or well is longer than in the original Jay cushions. This reduces bottoming out especially with clients who are sacral sitters. These clients usually slide forward in the wheelchair and hit the central slope of the base with the fluid migrating behind the buttocks. Similar to the original Jay cushions, the pelvis is positioned lower than the legs putting the hips into flexion and keeping the femurs parallel to the seat. This helps to stabilize the pelvis, decreasing the risk of sliding forward and out of the wheelchair and providing trunk stability. The contoured base has sculptured leg channels which encourage a neutral leg position. Since it is firm, the solid base can overhang the sling seat by 5 cm (2 in.) thus allowing the use of a longer cushion to accommodate, for example, the thigh length of taller clients. The bottom of the contoured base is non-skid to help prevent the cushion from sliding on the wheelchair seat.

The J-2 cushion comes with a slip-on cover. The top part is made of a tough stretch material with a durable ballistic material around the edges. The cushion is easy to clean and needs to be stored flat.

Assembly:

See page 45 (Pelvis, Jay Cushions). Unlike the Jay cushions, the J-2 cushion contoured base does not require painting to seal the surface after cuts and modifications.

Jay Care Cushion (Jay Medical Ltd)

The Jay Care cushion is a positioning and pressure relief cushion designed specifically for the older adult or for the individual whose sensation is intact but who is at risk for skin breakdown. The Jay Care cushion is a sealed unit made of a soft contoured foam cushion with a moisture-proof casing. The foam cushion is contoured to provide leg channels and a slight backward angle, or pre-ischial bar. This stabilizes the pelvis, prevents sliding forward and out of the wheelchair, and promotes a neutral leg position, i.e., maintaining the femurs parallel to the seat and to each other. The foam base has a reinforced curved bottom to help counteract the effect of the sling seat providing a level sitting base for the pelvis and the lower extremities. The foam base has a non-skid bottom to prevent movement of the cushion in the wheelchair. The moisture-proof casing is segmented and contains the built-in Jay flow fluid which provides pressure relief. The Jay flow is maintenance free, i.e., does not require regular kneading, and maintains its viscosity at high and low temperatures. The cover of the Jay Care cushion is made of washable stretch material.

The Jay Care cushion is intended to be used primarily in conjunction with the Jay care back to create the Jay Care seating system; see page 106 (Trunk, Jay Care Back). It helps solve common seating problems resulting from the wheelchair sling seat and back. The Jay Care seating system is designed to position the pelvis and the lower extremities, to prevent sliding forward and out of the wheelchair, to promote good alignment of the spine, and to accommodate a mild to moderate kyphotic posture (Figure 5-16).

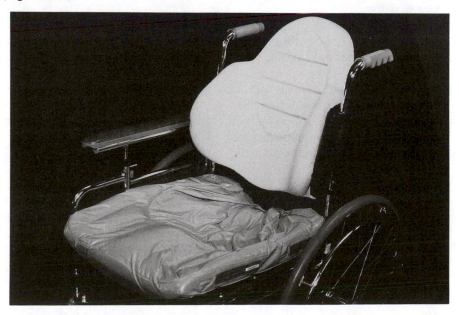

Figure 5-16. Jay Care seating system.

The Jay Care cushion is available in two standard widths: 45 and 40 cm (18 and 16 in.) and two standard depths: 40 and 45 cm (16 and 18 in.).

Assembly:

The Jay Care cushion is ready to use and requires no maintenance. Because of the curved bottom, the Jay Care cushion can be used on a sling seat or on a dropped solid seat. If the sling seat is overly stretched, i.e., more than 6 cm (2.5 in.) from the seat rail level to the lowest point of the sling seat, replacement of the sling seat is recommended. The Jay Care cushion can overhang the sling seat by 5 cm (2 in.), i.e., 2.5 cm (1 in.) at the front and the same at the back.

Since the Jay Care cushion is one sealed solid unit, cuts to modify the shape of the cushion are not possible.

Level Base of Support

A level base of support is necessary to counteract the hammock effect of the sling seat. It prevents pelvic obliquity thus helping to distribute the pressure evenly under both buttocks and can also assist in the prevention of upper body leaning. A level base of support helps to prevent sacral sitting and promotes neutral rotation at the hips with a neutral leg position.

The following four methods provide a level base of support. Because they are placed on top of the sling seat, they increase the height of the sitting surface. This can become either an advantage, for example, to the tall client in getting his or her feet off the ground, or a disadvantage to the short client as standing transfers may be more difficult.

Plywood Board

Construction:

1. A board of 1 cm (3/8 in.) plywood (Figure 5-17) is cut to fit the size of the wheelchair seat. The corners are rounded.
2. The board is placed on top of the sling seat and must be supported on the two seat rails.
3. The board should be tied to the back frame of the wheelchair by drilling two holes in the back corners and attaching ties.
4. A cushion is placed on the plywood. It can be fixed to the plywood with Velcro to prevent the cushion from sliding forward or backward. The foam and cover can be stapled to the plywood board.

Wedge Board With Foam Cushion

The wedge board with foam cushion is recommended to prevent mild to moderate problems of sacral sitting and sliding. The addition of the board will also provide a firm sitting surface to prevent pelvic obliquity.

More often used when positioning a client in a reclining wheelchair, a wedge board with foam cushion helps to maintain hip flexion at about 100 degrees.

The wedge board should be tied to the back frame of the wheelchair to prevent it from sliding forward with the client.

The height of the footrests should be adjusted to accommodate the increased seat height caused by the wedge.

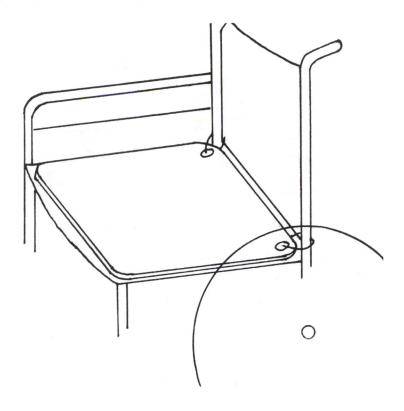

Figure 5-17. Plywood board.

Construction:
1. The board is made of 0.6 cm (0.25 in.) plywood and 1.2 cm (1 in.) plywood.
2. Cut two pieces of 0.6 cm (0.25 in.) plywood the same width and depth as the wheelchair seat.
3. Cut one piece of the 1.2 cm (1 in.) plywood the width of the wheelchair seat. The height depends on the height required at the front of the wedge which is usually 3 cm (1.25 in.) high for a wedge board with cushion of 7.5 cm (3 in.) high. Cut another length 2 cm (1.75 in.) high.
4. The wedge board is assembled according to Figure 5-18. All the pieces are glued and nailed together.
5. The wedge board is varnished for cleanliness.
6. A cushion is cut out of 7.5 cm (3 in.) medium density foam to fit the size of the wedge board.
7. The cover is made with a durable and stretchable fabric. The cover and foam cushion are stapled to the wedge board to prevent the cushion from sliding forward.

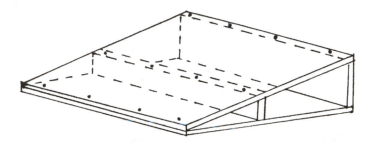

Figure 5-18. Wedge board.

Champher Foam Base

A champher foam base is a cushion which is thick in the middle and thin on each side. It is an alternative way to provide a level base of support. Unlike the plywood board, the champher foam base tends to move less in the wheelchair as it fills the sag of the sling seat. If the client bottoms out on a 5 or 7.5 cm (2 or 3 in.) foam cushion, the champher foam base is a softer option than using a board to provide a level surface.

Made of extra firm chip foam, the champher foam base can overhang the sling seat depth thus accommodating a client who requires a deeper seat.

Construction:

1. A champher foam base is made of extra firm chip foam or reconstituted polyether foam.
2. The foam base is cut to fit the width and depth of the sling seat. It is 5 cm (2 in.) thick in the middle tapering to 0 on each side (Figure 5-19). To provide a longer seat base, 2.5 to 5 cm (1 to 2 in.) can be added to the measurement of the seat depth. Rounding the back of the champher foam base from side to side fills the gap between the back of the sling seat and the back canvas. It also prevents the champher from sliding back on the seat or the seat cushion protruding behind the back canvas.
3. The champher foam base is covered with non-skid material. Ties are sewn in all four corners to secure the base to the wheelchair.

QA2 Seat Base (QA2 Seating System)

The QA2 seat base (Figure 5-20) is made of strong ABS thermal plastic. The seat base inserts on the wheelchair seat rails with no modification to the wheelchair.

The QA2 seat base can be fitted to most types of standard adult and reclining wheelchairs with widths ranging from 36 to 51 cm (14 to 20 in.) and of varying seat depths.

QA2 flat or wedge cushions are available and are secured to the seat base with Velcro. The wedge cushion is 7.5 cm (3 in.) thick at the front and 5 cm (2 in.) thick at the back. Cushions are made of medium density foam with a water-resistant Ultraskin cover.

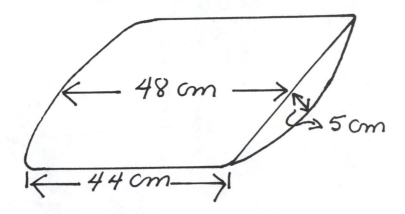

Figure 5-19. Champher foam base.

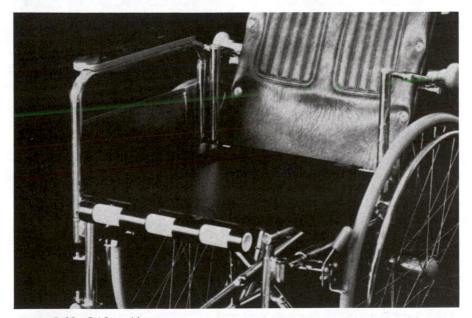

Figure 5-20. QA2 seat base.

SHS Cushion (Special Health Systems)

The SHS cushion (Figure 5-21) fits the contour of the sling seat and provides a level sitting surface. There are two types of SHS cushions: one for standard seating requirements and one for sensitive seating requirements. The SHS cushion comes in standard or wedge (2.5 cm or 1 in. lower at the back).

Standard SHS cushions are made of 2.5 or 5 cm (1 or 2 in.) medium density foam

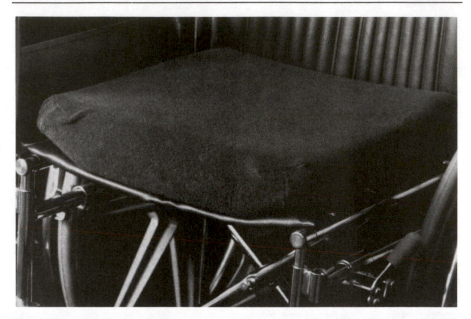

Figure 5-21. SHS cushion.

and 2.5 cm (1 in.) comfort foam. Cushions for sensitive seating requirements have an extra 2.5 cm (1 in.) contouring foam.

The cushions are covered with a durable and waterproof stretch neoprene cover. An outer covering is available in stretch terry cloth.

The SHS cushions are 43.5 x 43.5 cm (17 x 17 in.) to fit narrow and regular adult wheelchair sling seats.

Drop Seat Base

A drop seat base can be used with any type of cushion to prevent build-up of the height of the seat and to provide a level base of support.

Various problems may be created by a seat which is too high:

• Mobilization of the wheelchair with the lower extremities becomes difficult or impossible.

• Transferring may become hazardous.

• Armrests and back height may be too low thus affecting trunk stability.

• Environmental difficulties such as being unable to get the knees under a table often occur.

Wooden Drop Seat

The wooden drop seat (Figure 5-22) lowers the seating surface by 5 cm (2 in.). Lowering a seat more than 5 cm (2 in.) below the seat rails is not advisable. The crossbars will press against the lateral aspect of the thighs and become a source of discomfort and a potential site of pressure sores.

Construction:

1. The wooden drop seat is made of 1 cm (3/8 in.) plywood and four stainless steel

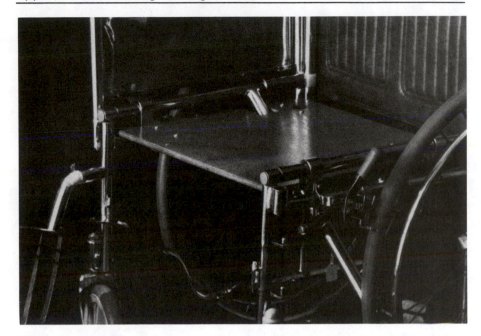

Figure 5-22. Wooden drop seat.

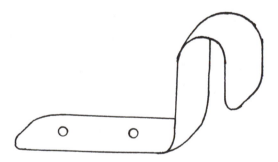

Figure 5-23. Suspension hook.

suspension hooks (wheelchair brackets, IDC Tectonics Ltd) (Figure 5-23).
2. For a 46 cm (18 in.) wide wheelchair with the sling seat removed cut a piece of plywood 40 cm (15.75 in.) long and 38.5 cm (15 in.) wide.
3. Two spaces 3 cm (1.25 in.) wide and 6 cm (2.5 in.) long are cut so the board will fit over the crossbars (see Figure 5-22).
4. The four suspension hooks are fixed to the board with bolts.

It is advisable to tie the drop seat to the wheelchair as the seat may tilt forward if the client slides forward in the wheelchair.

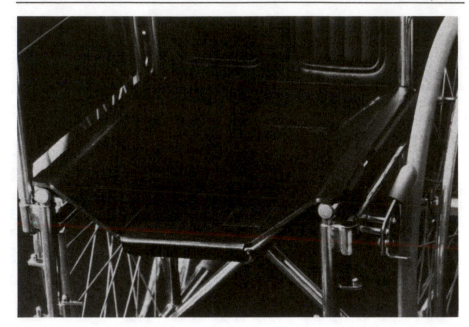

Figure 5-24. QA2 drop seat base.

QA2 Drop Seat Base (QA2 Seating System)

The QA2 drop seat base (Figure 5-24) can be fitted to most types of standard adult and reclining wheelchairs with widths from 36 to 46 cm (14 to 18 in.).

The ABS plastic molded seat base inserts onto the wheelchair seat rails with the sling seat removed. The drop seat base is secured to the wheelchair with two Velcro straps located under the seat base. It lowers the height of the seat by 6.5 cm (2.5 in.).

The drop seat base can be fitted with a QA2 flat cushion or a wedge cushion. The cushion is fixed to the drop seat base with Velcro. It is made of medium density foam with a water-resistant Ultraskin cover.

SHS Fiberglass Low Seat (Special Health Systems)

The SHS fiberglass low seat (Figure 5-25) can be fitted to most types of standard adult and reclining wheelchairs. It is available in one standard size: 46 cm (18 in.) wide.

With the sling seat removed, the molded fiberglass seat inserts onto the wheelchair seat rails. It lowers the seating surface by 6.5 cm (2.5 in.).

A compatible SHS low seat cushion made of 5 cm (2 in.) medium density foam with a neoprene shell and a stretch terry cloth cover can be used with the fiberglass low seat.

Jay Adjustable Solid Seat (Jay Medical Ltd)

The Jay adjustable solid seat (Figure 5-26) can be fitted to most types of wheelchairs with seat widths ranging from 38 to 46 cm (15 to 18 in.). The seat base is made of molded, reinforced urethane. Once the sling seat is removed, it is secured to the wheelchair seat rails with four steel hooks. A hook stopper fitted on the rail

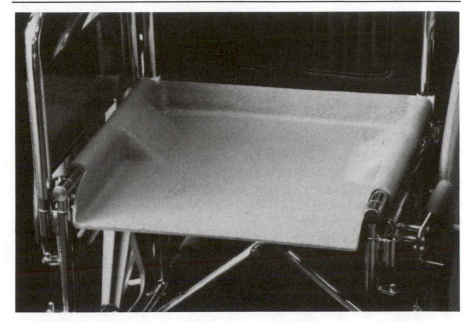

Figure 5-25. SHS fiberglass low seat.

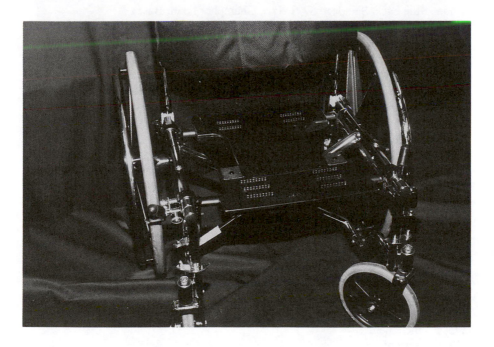

Figure 5-26. Jay adjustable solid seat.

prevents the seat from sliding forward. Two hook retainers prevent the seat from sliding backward or accidentally popping out of the wheelchair.

The Jay adjustable solid seat can be slid forward for a 46 cm (18 in.) seat depth or it can be cut down to a 31.5 cm (12 in.) length. The seat can be raised or lowered in 1.25 cm (0.5 in.) increments from 2.5 cm (1 in.) above the seat rails to 3.75 cm (1.5 in.) below the rails. It is also possible to angle the seat base by setting the hooks at different lengths at the front and back. Crossbar cut-outs on the base allow dropping the seat on most types of wheelchair.

Due to the ease of adjustment, all nuts and bolts on the Jay solid seat need to be checked on a regular basis and tightened as necessary.

Long Seat Base

Most types of wheelchairs have a standard seat depth of 41 cm (16 in.). This is limiting for taller clients who have a longer thigh length or require a longer sitting surface due to a fixed posterior pelvic tilt. An appropriate seat depth provides the client with the longest possible sitting base thus increasing stability in sitting and helping distribute the weight over the longest possible surface.

Wheelchairs can be ordered with a custom seat depth. For clients who own a wheelchair, other ways to create a longer seat base include:

- Champher foam base that overhangs the sling seat by 2.5 (1 in.) at the front and the same at the back. See page 52 (Pelvis, Champher Foam Base).
- Jay cushions (Jay Medical Ltd) which can overhang the sling seat by 2.5 to 5 cm (1 to 2 in.) See page 45 (Pelvis, Jay Cushions).
- Longer wooden drop seat base that is securely fastened in all four corners of the wheelchair frame. See page 54 (Pelvis, Wooden Drop Seat).
- Jay adjustable solid seat (Jay Medical Ltd) can be slid forward to create a seat depth of up to 46 cm (18 in.) See page 56 (Pelvis, Jay Adjustable Solid Seat).

Adjustable Suspension Hooks

Adjustable suspension hooks are used to make a wooden level seating surface which replaces the sling seat of the wheelchair. Depending on the length of the seat board, the seat depth can be shortened or lengthened. The adjustable suspension hooks allow raising, lowering, or wedging of the seating surface. For a description of the different applications of a level, dropped, wedged, or long seat base, see pages 50 (Pelvis, Level Base of Support), 54 (Pelvis, Drop Seat Base), and 58 (Pelvis, Long Seat Base).

The adjustable suspension hooks (Figure 5-27) are made in two parts and usually of stainless steel. They are available from various companies such as Avanti seating and positioning products (Invacare Corp). Hook adjustments usually range from 5.5 cm (2.25 in.) below the seat rails to 5.5 cm (2.25 in.) above the seat rails with 1.7 cm (0.75 in.) increments.

Construction:
1. Four adjustable suspension hooks are required to make a seat. The two parts of each adjustable suspension hook are fastened together using bolts, nuts, and lock washers. By using the different holes on the two parts of the adjustable suspension hook, a dropped, raised, or tilted seat can be created (see Figure 5-27).

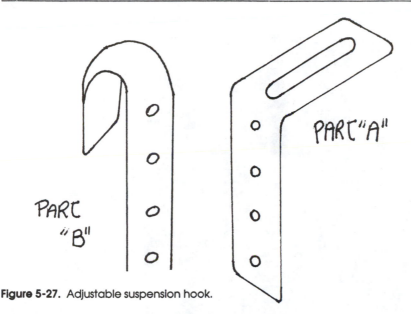

Figure 5-27. Adjustable suspension hook.

2. To measure and cut an appropriate wooden seat board to fit your client with cut-outs for the wheelchair crossbars, see pages 54 (Pelvis, Wooden Drop Seat) and 58 (Pelvis, Long Seat Base).
3. The wooden seat board is fixed to part "A" of the suspension hook (Figure 5-28) using bolts, nuts, and lock washers. The lengthwise opening in part "A" of the suspension hook is to allow minimal adjustment in the width of the seat.
4. With the sling seat removed, the wooden seat board is suspended on the wheelchair seat rails. The seat is secured in all four corners as the seat may tilt forward if the client slides forward in the wheelchair.

45 Degree Lap Belt (Special Health Systems)

The 45 degree angle lap belt (Figure 5-29) is used to prevent the pelvis from tilting backward and sliding forward in the wheelchair.

The lap belt will restrain the client from transferring independently or repositioning in the wheelchair, so it should be used only if sacral sitting and sliding cannot be prevented by positioning with a cushion, for example.

An appropriate cushion (one of the types recommended for sacral sitting) should be used in conjunction with the lap belt.

A 45 degree angle lap belt can be fitted to any type of adult wheelchair.

Assembly:

The SHS 45 degree angle lap belt is made of 5 cm (2 in.) wide nylon webbing with a lightweight plastic buckle at the front.

It is secured with the back screws on the seat rails of the wheelchair. The lap belt is positioned over but not above the iliac crests (hip bone) and at a 45 degree angle. If the lap belt is positioned above the iliac crests, it will pull the pelvis into a posterior tilt. For a client with a fixed posterior pelvic tilt, the lap belt can be

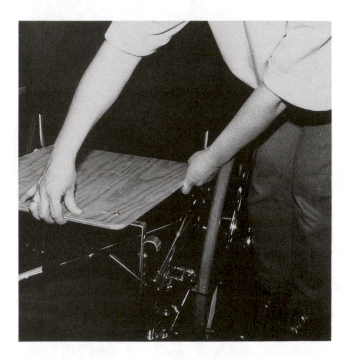

Figure 5-28. Tilted drop seat base.

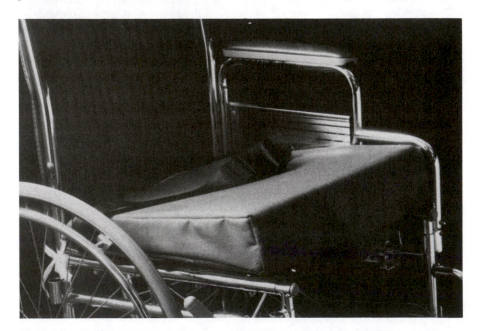

Figure 5-29. 45 degree lap belt.

positioned over the iliac crests at a 60 degree angle by securing it further forward on the seat rails of the wheelchair. The lap belt should fit snugly but comfortably.

Other types of seat belts should be positioned on the wheelchair in the same way.

Lower Extremities

The thighs and pelvis are the sitting base or base of support. The position and alignment of the femurs play a major role in stabilizing the pelvis in a slightly tilted forward position. The feet resting flat on the footrests bring stability to the sitting base, prevent sliding forward in the wheelchair, and facilitate repositioning of self in the wheelchair. Balance and freedom of movement of the upper body are directly related to the stability of the lower body.

Potential Problems
- One or both feet fall off the footrest/legrest. They may fall behind, to the side, or in front of the footrest. The feet may be injured by the front casters or they may drag on the floor.
    - This may be due to hypotonicity, hypertonicity, or weakness of one or both lower extremities.
    - Hypertonicity of the flexor muscles of the knees or flexion contractures will limit the ability to extend the knees beyond 90 degrees to keep the feet flat on the foot plates. Hypertonicity or shortening of the hamstring muscles also limits the ability to extend the knees. Mobilizing a wheelchair over rough or uneven terrain tends to stimulate an increase in flexor or extensor tone and a tremor which limits the ability to keep the feet flat on the foot plates.
    - The client may be unable to alert the caregiver or unable to independently lift the foot back onto the footrest. A lack of awareness of body position or impaired sensitivity will contribute to the problem.
- Lack of comfortable support for the foot caused by a foot plate that is too low.
- Lack of comfortable support for the foot caused by a foot plate that is too short. This can lead to a plantar flexion contracture deformity and the foot falling in front of the footplate.
- Presence of a positive support reflex as evidence by an increase in the extensor tone of the hip, knee, and ankle when the ball of the foot touches the foot plate. To inhibit this reflex, the foot needs full contact on the foot plate.
- Ankle clonus usually triggered when only the ball of the foot is in contact with the foot plate. To inhibit this reflex, the foot needs full contact on the foot plate and the ankle is positioned in a neutral position or slight dorsiflexion.
- Pain or discomfort for the client with above or below knee amputation usually caused by a lack of support to the amputated extremity. The end of the stump requires protection when the client is mobilizing in a wheelchair. For the below knee amputee, contractures of the knee and dependent edema must be prevented if the client wears a prosthesis.
- Edema. Swelling that is present in the ankle and the foot and may extend up the calf.

- Injury of the lower extremities through uncontrolled movements such as spasms or from a lack of awareness of body position.
- An open sore on the lateral aspect of the knee that is caused by pressure against the raised pivot point of the elevating legrest.
- Hypertonicity of hip adductors causing the thighs to roll in and the knees to press together. This results in increased pressure on the medial aspect of the knees and the risk of a pressure sore. It also reduces the rectangular shape of the sitting surface created by the pelvis and the thighs to a less stable triangular shape. The subsequent difficulty in balancing the long unstable column of the trunk over the smaller base leads to poor trunk control and limited sitting balance. Adduction of the lower extremities can be compounded or actively promoted by a sagging seat canvas.
- Wind swept deformity, one hip abducted and one hip adducted causing the legs to appear unequal in length. Since this is a complex problem, various factors such as rotation of the pelvis, pelvic obliquity, muscle imbalance, and/or short wheelchair seat depth may cause this deformity. See page 35 (Pelvis, "Wind Swept" Deformity).

Special Considerations
- Transfer modality. The method used to transfer the client from the wheelchair to the bed will affect the choice of positioning device. A legrest cradle, for example, may prevent the clients legs from falling off the footrests but a standing pivot transfer will be difficult for the client and the caregiver.
- Changing the center of gravity of a wheelchair by fully elevating both legrests may be hazardous. A standard frame wheelchair cannot always accommodate the extra weight at the front especially if the client is tall and/or heavy. The wheelchair may easily tip forward. This can be prevented by adding anti-tipping weights at the back of the wheelchair or by using a reclining wheelchair.

Possible Solutions
- Elevating blocks on foot plates
- Foot plate extension
- Knee protector for elevating legrests
- Heel strap
- Legrest panel
    Fabric legrest panel
    Legrest panel—one piece hook-on leatherette (Everest and Jennings)
- Foot support
    Wooden foot support
    SHS foot support kit (Special Health Systems)
- Wooden foot support with posterior extension
- Board support on legrests
    Legrest board
    Leg and footrest board
- Padded wooden legrest
- Amputee cushion

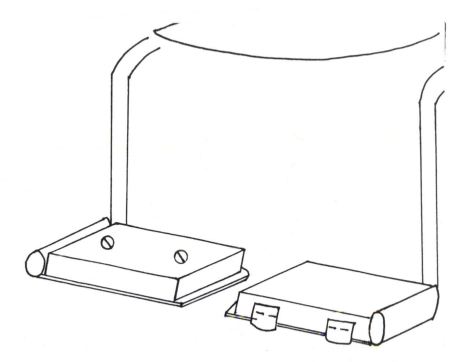

Figure 5-30. Elevating blocks fixed with bolts (left) and wide elastic strap (right).

- Foot strap
     Figure "8" foot strap
     Ankle strap
- Ankle positioning aids
     Ankle positioning blocks
     Foot plates with adjustable angle setting (Everest and Jennings)
- Knee abductor

Elevating Blocks on Foot Plates

If the foot plates are raised to their shortest position and the client's feet still are not supported on the foot plates, comfortable support can be provided through the use of elevating blocks (Figure 5-30).

Construction:
1. Elevating blocks are made of 5 x 15 cm (2 x 6 in.) lumber cut to fit the size of the foot plate.
2. To confirm the height of the foot plate slip two fingers under the thigh to a depth of approximately 3.75 to 5 cm (1.5 to 2 in.) or check that the femurs are parallel to the seat and the full length of the thighs are supported on the cushion.
3. Secure the block to the foot plate with two bolts. The block and the foot plate are drilled and the nut is screwed under the foot plate.
4. Another method of securing the block to the foot plate is with an elastic strap. A

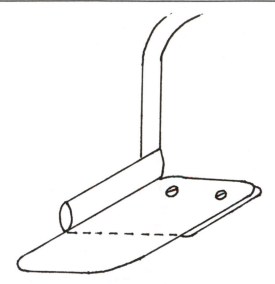

Figure 5-31. Foot plate extension.

5 cm (2 in.) wide strip of elastic is stapled to the two sides of the block and loops under the foot plate. The first method of securing the block is preferable as it is a more permanent solution.

Foot Plate Extension

Foot plate extensions are fitted on top of existing foot plates to increase the length of the foot plate (Figure 5-31).

Foot plates that are too short can cause serious problems for the client with high tone, spasms, or tremors. The feet tend to fall in front of the footrests. This can lead to plantar flexion deformities. Sitting balance and stability are compromised as the client cannot rely on the support provided by the feet resting flat on the foot plates to prevent sliding forward in the wheelchair. It also makes it more difficult to push oneself back up in the wheelchair. The ability to do a standing transfer or to ambulate can be jeopardized.

Construction:
1. Foot plate extensions are made of 0.5 cm (0.25 in.) plywood cut to fit the width of the foot plate.
2. To determine the length, measure the length of the foot 2.5 cm (1 in.) from the heel to the metatarsophalangeal joints. Foot plate extensions can be made longer but the extra length adds to the overall length of the wheelchair and may pose environmental problems.
3. Corners are rounded and the foot plate extensions are covered with non-skid material.
4. Two holes are drilled in the extension and the foot plate. Secure the extension to the foot plate with two bolts. The nuts are screwed under the foot plate.

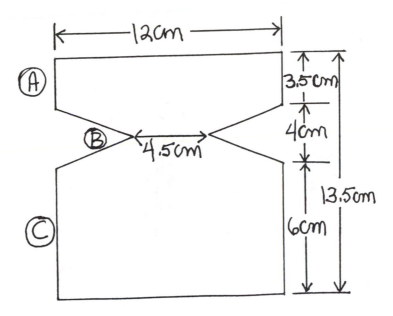

Figure 5-32. Diagram of knee protector.

Knee Protector for Elevating Legrests

When using elevating legrests the lateral aspect of the knee may press against the raised pivot point of the legrest. This area is at risk for the development of a pressure sore and is often a source of discomfort.

Construction:

1. The knee protector is made of 1.2 cm (0.5 in.) low temperature closed-cell foam such as plastazote which is cut as shown in Figure 5-32.
2. Mold the plastazote around the raised pivot point of the hinge. To position refer to Figure 5-32. "A" is the top section and "C" is the bottom section. Bend at "B" over the pivot point.
3. The knee protector (Figure 5-33) is held in place with 2.5 cm (1 in.) wide Velcro straps.

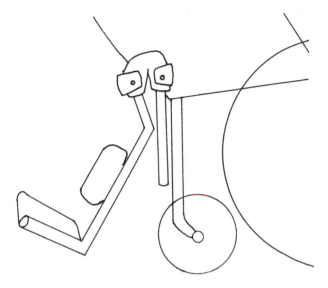

Figure 5-33. Knee protector.

Heel Strap

The heel strap (Figure 5-34) is used to prevent the feet from falling off the back of the footrests.

When increased tone in the flexor muscles of the lower extremities is the cause of this problem, the heel strap is not recommended because the feet will probably rise over the heel strap and get caught behind the footrest.

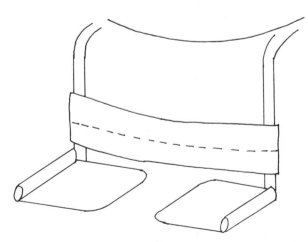

Figure 5-34. Heel strap.

Construction:

1. The heel strap is made of a strong durable material such as leather or webbing approximately 7.5 to 10 cm (3 to 4 in.) wide. Two lengths of webbing can be sewn together if necessary.
2. The strap is long enough to wrap around the footrest and overlap by 10 to 12.5 cm (4 to 5 in.). The heel strap is secured using Velcro.

Legrest Panel

The legrest panel prevents the lower extremities from falling between and behind the footrests.

It is recommended for use with clients who have increased tone in the flexor muscles of the lower extremities but only when they are able to extend their knees beyond 90 degrees to rest their feet flat on the footrests. It can also be used for clients who have weakness or lack of awareness of their lower extremities.

The legrest panel can be used with footrests or with elevating legrests.

Fabric Legrest Panel
Construction:

1. Use a durable material such as leatherette or denim.
2. To fit a 41 or 46 cm (16 or 18 in.) wide adult wheelchair, cut a piece of material 28 cm (11 in.) long and 43 cm (17 in.) wide (Figure 5-35).
3. Four lengths of 5 cm (2 in.) wide Velcro are sewn, one in each corner, to attach the legrest panel to the footrest. A 7 cm (2.5 in.) strip of hook Velcro is sewn on the corner of the panel with the adjoining 15 cm (6 in.) strip of loop Velcro (Figure 5-36).

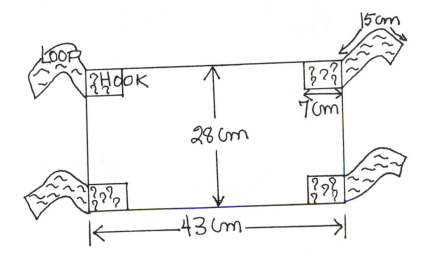

Figure 5-35. Diagram of fabric legrest panel.

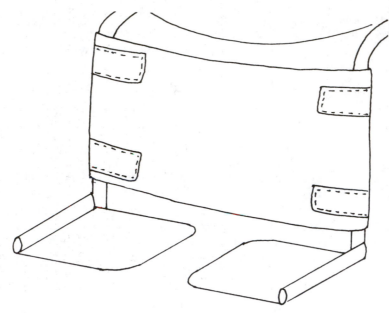

Figure 5-36. Fabric legrest panel.

Legrest Panel—One Piece Hook-On Leatherette (Everest and Jennings)

Assembly:

This leatherette legrest panel is useful with elevating legrests or footrests. It easily attaches to the legrests with four metal hooks (Figure 5-37).

It is not appropriate for clients who have severe hypertonicity of the flexor muscles of the lower extremities because the metal hooks may be stretched by the constant leg pressure against the panel. Standard widths available are 41 and 46 cm (16 and 18 in.).

Foot Support

The foot support prevents the feet from falling between or behind the foot plates and is used with clients who have hypotonicity, weakness, or mild increase in extensor tone of one or both lower extremities. It is also useful in preventing foot injury for clients who have poor body awareness. It provides good support for the whole length of the foot. The foot support can be mounted on footrests or elevating legrests. It is secured to only one foot plate which permits it to swing away with the footrest for ease of transfer.

Wooden Foot Support

Construction:

1. Use 0.6 cm (0.25 in.) plywood.
2. To fit a 46 cm (18 in.) wide adult wheelchair, cut the following pieces as shown in Figure 5-38.
3. Pieces 1 and 2 are fixed together at 90 degrees with two 5 cm (2 in.) long corner

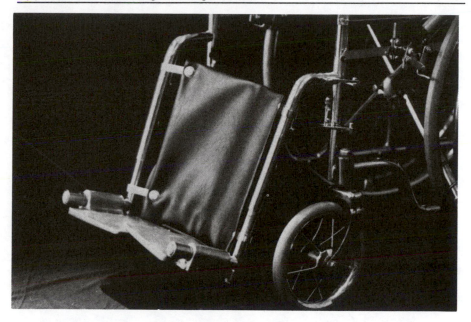

Figure 5-37. Everest and Jennings legrest panel.

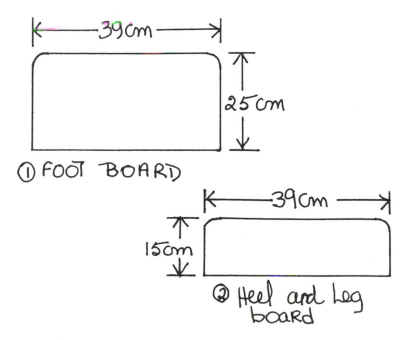

Figure 5-38. Diagram of wooden support boards.

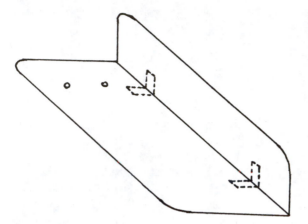

Figure 5-39. Foot support.

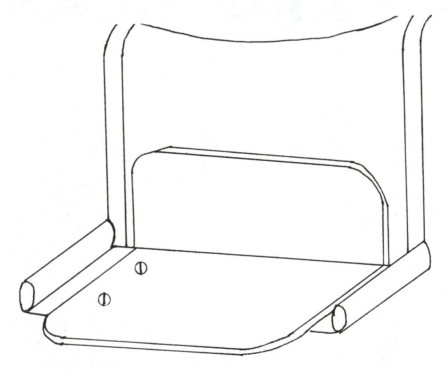

Figure 5-40. Wooden foot support.

braces and bolts (Figure 5-39).
4. Two holes are drilled in one side of the foot board to align with two holes drilled in one of the foot plates.
5. The wooden foot support can be either varnished or padded with 2.5 cm (1 in.) low density foam covered with a durable fabric such as denim.

6. The wooden foot support is secured to one foot plate with two bolts (Figure 5-40).

SHS Foot Support Kit (Special Health Systems)

Assembly:

The foot support kit is made of strong thermoplastic material. It is mounted on the right foot plate extending across the left foot plate to provide support for both feet (Figure 5-41).

The foot support swings away with the footrest for ease of transfer. It can be fitted to 41 or 46 cm (16 or 18 in.) wide wheelchairs.

Wooden Foot Support With Posterior Extension

The wooden foot support with posterior extension prevents the feet from falling between and behind the foot plates. It is used with clients who have hypertonicity of the flexor muscles of the knees or flexion contractures which limit extension to 90 degrees maximum but not less than 75 degrees.

It provides good support for the whole length of the foot. The foot support is mounted on the footrests. It is secured to only one foot plate which permits it to swing away with the footrest for ease of transfer.

Construction:

1. Use 0.6 cm (0.25 in.) plywood and 2.5 x 2.5 cm (1 x 1 in.) wooden strip.
2. To fit a 46 cm (18 in.) wide adult wheelchair, cut the following pieces as shown in Figure 5-42.
3. The spaces marked "A" on the foot board are to allow the front casters to swing freely (see Figure 5-42).

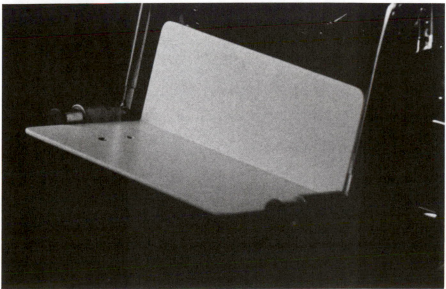

Figure 5-41. SHS foot support kit.

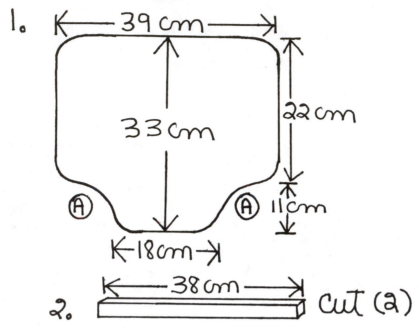

Figure 5-42. Diagram of foot support.

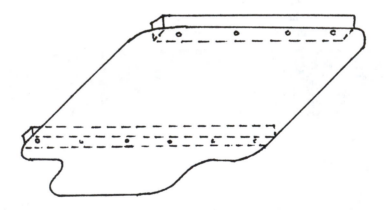

Figure 5-43. Stopper placement on wooden foot support with posterior extension.

4. One stopper is fixed under the foot board with glue and screws (Figure 5-43). It is situated in front of the foot plates to prevent the board from moving behind them.

5. One stopper is fixed under the foot board with glue and screws to sit on the posterior part of the foot plates. This is to keep the foot board level (see Figure 5-43).

6. Two holes are drilled in one side of the foot board to align with two holes drilled on one of the foot plates.

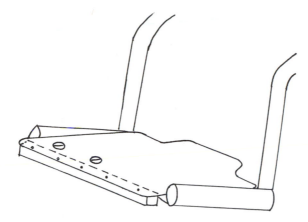

Figure 5-44. Wooden foot support with posterior extension.

7. The wooden foot support with posterior extension can be either varnished or padded with 2.5 cm (1 in.) low density foam and covered with a durable fabric such as denim.
8. The foot board extension is secured to one foot plate with two bolts. The nuts are situated under the foot plate (Figure 5-44).

Board Support on Legrests

The board support is intended to provide support to the lower extremities and prevent them from falling between or behind elevating legrests. This support can also be used with clients who have a below knee amputation.

A foot board can be added to provide support to the feet. It is convenient with clients who transfer with a mechanical lift as the board does not have to be removed during transfer.

Legrest Board
Construction:
1. Use 0.5 cm (0.25 in.) plywood.
2. To determine the width of the board required, measure the distance between the legrests within the posts. For example, for a 46 cm (18 in.) wide adult wheelchair use a board 39 cm (15.5 in.) wide.
3. The length depends on the client's leg length. Measure from just below the raised pivot point on the legrest to the bottom of the client's calf.
4. The corners of the board are rounded and two holes 2 cm (0.75 in.) diameter are drilled in the upper corners.
5. The board is padded with 2.5 cm (1 in.) low density foam and covered with a soft, durable fabric. The cover is stapled to the back of the board.
6. Two 2.5 cm (1 in.) wide Velcro straps secured to the holes attach the legrest board to the wheelchair (Figure 5-45).

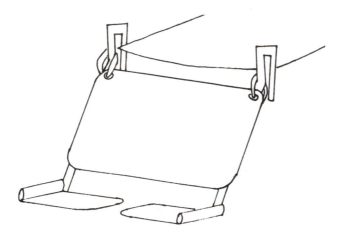

Figure 5-45. Legrest board.

Construction:
1. Use 0.5 cm (0.25 in.) plywood.
2. To determine the width of the board, measure the distance between the legrests within the posts. For example, for a 46 cm (18 in.) wide adult wheelchair use a board 39 cm (15.5 in.) wide.
3. The length of the board depends on the client's leg length. Measure from just below the raised pivot point on the legrest to the client's heel with the ankle at 90 degrees or to the toes if the client has a drop foot. Add 2.5 cm (1 in.) to that measurement.
4. The top two corners of the board are rounded. Four holes 2 cm (0.75 in.) are drilled: two in the upper corners and one on each side halfway down the board (Figure 5-46).
5. The foot board is cut the same width as the leg board. The height of the board is determined by adding 5 cm (2 in.) to the length of the client's foot. The two top corners are rounded (see Figure 5-46).
6. The leg board and foot board are secured together at 90 degrees using two corner

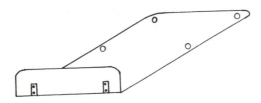

Figure 5-46. Leg and footrest board.

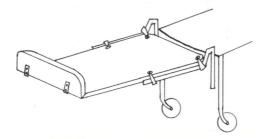

Figure 5-47. Leg and footrest board.

braces 5 cm (2 in.) long and 2 cm (0.75 in.) long bolts.
7. The board is padded with a 2.5 cm (1 in.) low density foam and covered with a soft, durable fabric. The cover is stapled to the back of the board.
8. Four 2.5 cm (1 in.) Velcro straps attach through the holes to secure the board to the legrests (Figure 5-47). The wheelchair foot plates can be removed if necessary.

Padded Wooden Legrest

The padded wooden legrest provides additional protection and support for one lower extremity on an elevating legrest. It prevents the leg from falling off the elevating legrest and provides a larger area of support.

The padded wooden legrest can be fitted to any type of elevating legrest. It does not interfere with the client's ability to transfer as it is attached to the mounting bracket of the standard legrest panel and can be swung away.

Construction:
1. Use 1 cm (3/8 in.) plywood.
2. Cut two pieces of plywood:
   • 35 x 7.5 cm (14 x 3 in.)
   • 35 x 18 cm (14 x 7 in.)
   • Round the corners (Figure 5-48)
3. The pieces are joined at a right angle with two 4 cm (1.5 in.) long corner braces and bolts.
4. The original legrest panel is removed from the elevating legrest and the wooden legrest is secured to the mounting bracket with bolts.
5. The wooden legrest is padded with 2.5 cm (1 in.) low density foam.
6. It can be covered with any soft, durable fabric. The cover is stapled to the padded wooden legrest (Figure 5-49).

Amputee Cushion

The amputee cushion is a padded wooden seat base plus a padded board that inserts into the seat base. It will provide support and protection for the stump, for example, when going through a narrow doorway.

The amputee cushion with stump board is also used in the treatment of a client with a below knee amputation in the pre-prosthetic stage. By supporting the stump,

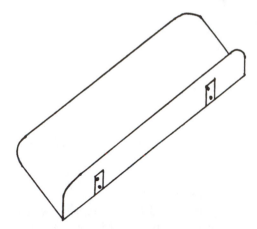

Figure 5-48. Wooden legrest.

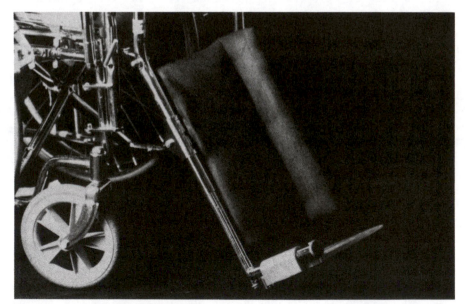

Figure 5-49. Padded wooden legrest.

the board will prevent the development of a flexion contracture in the knee. As well, it will prevent the formation of dependent edema which would retard wound healing or increase the risk of skin breakdown. This would result in delay for prosthetic fitting. The padded board is removable for when the client is wearing a prothesis or to permit transferring.

The amputee cushion can be constructed for any type of standard adult or reclining wheelchair.

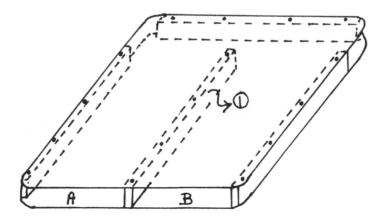

Figure 5-50. Seat base.

Construction:
1. The amputee cushion is made of 0.6 cm (0.25 in.) plywood.
2. Cut two seat boards the size of the wheelchair seat. The pieces should be wide enough to sit on the wheelchair seat rails. The corners are rounded.
3. Cut four pieces of 1 cm (3/8 in.) plywood 1 cm (3/8 in.) wide. Three of the pieces are the same length as the depth of the seat boards minus 2.5 cm (1 in.). One piece is the same length as the width of the seat boards minus 2.5 cm (1 in.).
4. The two seat boards and the four plywood strips are assembled according to Figure 5-50. They are secured with glue and screws. Piece 1 is secured in the center of the seat base.
5. The amputee board is made of 0.6 cm (0.25 in.) plywood. To determine the width of the board, divide the width of the seat base by two and subtract 2 cm (0.75 in.). To calculate the length of the board, with the client sitting in the wheelchair, measure the length of the stump that is not supported on the seat base plus 3 cm (1.5 in.). The amputee board inserts in space "A" or "B" (see Figure 5-50), depending on the side of the amputation.
6. The seat base is padded with 5 cm (2 in.) medium density foam. The section of the amputee board that protrudes from the base is padded with the same foam. The foam is covered with any durable and stretchable fabric. It is stapled to the bottom of the seat base and the amputee board (Figure 5-51).

Foot Strap
A foot strap is used to prevent the foot from falling in front of the footrest due to hypotonicity, mild to moderate increased extensor tone, tremor, spasm, or a lack of body awareness. Increased extensor tone, tremor, or spasm is often stimulated when making an intense effort such as mobilizing the wheelchair, trying to push back up in the wheelchair when sliding forward, or when mobilizing the wheelchair over rough ground.

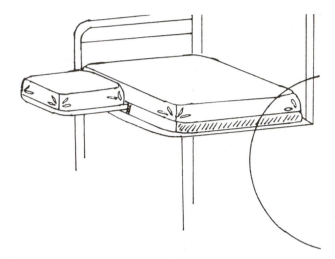

Figure 5-51. Above knee amputee cushion.

A short foot plate is often a contributing factor to this problem as it offers limited support to the foot and encourages plantar flexion. Check the foot plate length for adequate foot support. If a longer foot plate is required, see page 64 (Lower Extremities, Foot Plate Extension).

A foot strap is effective in maintaining the foot on the foot plate with the ankle at 90 degrees. It can also assist in preventing a plantar flexion contracture. A foot strap is not recommended if the foot slips off the foot plate due to a plantar flexion deformity and if adequate contact and support to the foot are not provided. See page 79 (Lower Extremities, Ankle Positioning Aids).

Foot straps can be fitted to most types of footrests or legrests.

Figure ''8'' Foot Strap
Construction:
1. Use 5 cm (2 in.) wide webbing, Velcro, and elastic.
2. Cut the following pieces:
   - Two lengths of webbing 22 cm (8.5 in.) long
   - One length of webbing 45 cm (18 in.) long
   - Two lengths of elastic 23 cm (9 in.) long
   - Two lengths of Velcro hook and loop each 9 cm (3.5 in.) long
3. Sew all the pieces together according to Figure 5-52. The end result should resemble the foot strap in Figure 5-53.

Ankle Strap
Construction:
1. Use 5 cm (2 in.) wide webbing, Velcro, and one "D" ring.
2. Cut a length of webbing 60 cm (24 in.) long and two lengths of Velcro hook and loop each 9 cm (3.5 in.) long.
3. Sew the pieces together according to Figure 5-54.

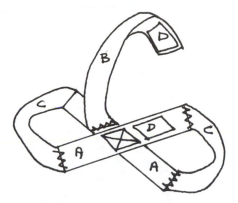

Figure 5-52. Left figure "8" foot strap.

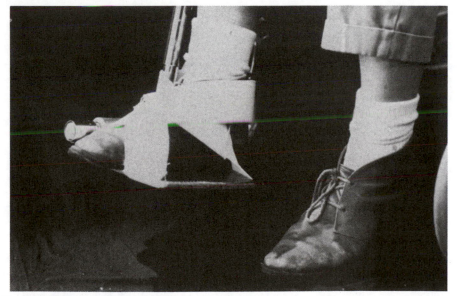

Figure 5-53. Figure "8" foot strap.

4. Two holes are drilled in the foot plate 2.5 cm (1 in.) from the back, 7.5 cm (3 in.) apart, and in the center of the foot plate (Figure 5-55).
5. The ankle strap is positioned on the foot plate so the "D" ring is situated on the lateral aspect of the foot (Figure 5-56).
6. The ankle strap is fixed to the foot plate with two nuts, bolts, and washers. The washer is situated on top of the strap. The nuts are situated under the foot plate.
7. A sleeve made of sheepskin can be slipped over the end of the strap which covers the foot for added comfort.

Ankle Positioning Aids
Ankle positioning aids are primarily designed for clients who have plantar flexion

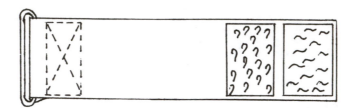

Figure 5-54. Ankle strap.

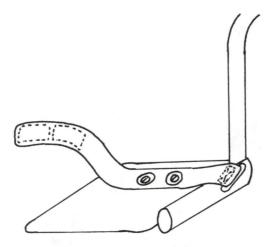

Figure 5-55. Left ankle strap.

contractures of the ankle. They are also used for clients who sit in a reclining wheelchair and who need extra foot support to maintain the ankle at 90 degrees.

They provide support for the whole length of the foot by adapting to the degree of ankle dorsiflexion required. Thus they improve the position of the lower extremities and sitting stability.

Ankle Positioning Blocks

Various types of lumber can be used to make the ankle positioning blocks (Figure 5-57) depending on the height required.

Ankle positioning blocks can be fitted to any type of footrest or elevating legrest.

Construction:

1. The length and width of the block is the same as the length and width of the foot plate.
2. The thin edge of the wedge should be approximately 0.5 cm (0.25 in.).
3. To determine the height of the thick edge of the wedge:
   - For a plantar flexion contracture: with the toes on the foot plate and the ankle in as much dorsiflexion as is comfortable, measure the distance from the heel to the foot plate.
   - To maintain a neutral ankle position: with the heel resting on the foot plate and

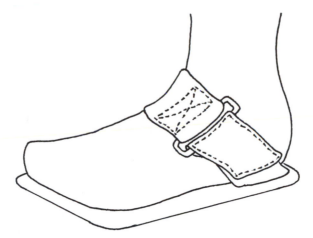

Figure 5-56. Left ankle strap.

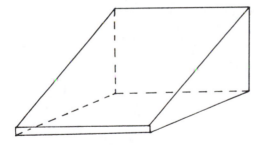

Figure 5-57. Ankle positioning block.

the ankle at 90 degrees, measure the distance between the toes and the foot plate.

4. The ankle positioning blocks are bolted to the foot plate (Figure 5-58).

5. The height of the footrest may need to be adjusted.

Foot Plates With Adjustable Angle Setting (Everest and Jennings)
Assembly:

Foot plates with an adjustable angle setting (Figure 5-59) can be fitted to any type of Everest and Jennings legrest or footrest. They may be adapted to other types of wheelchairs depending on the tubing size and method of attachment of the foot plate to the footrest.

The foot plates adjust to varying degrees of dorsiflexion or plantar flexion. The knob on the side of the foot plate adjusts the angle.

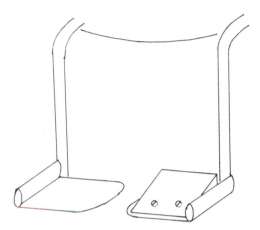

Figure 5-58. Fastened ankle positioning block.

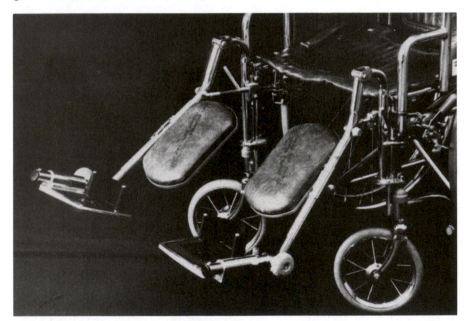

Figure 5-59. Foot plates with adjustable angle setting.

Knee Abductor

The knee abductor is used for clients who have increased tone in the adductor muscles of the thigh. It helps to minimize adduction contractures and pressure sores on the medial aspect of the knees. The knee abductor helps maintain the hips in neutral rotation, aligns the thighs parallel to each other, and keeps the pelvis level in order to maintain a wide base of support and a stable sitting posture.

Before fitting a client with a knee abductor, check the following points. First, ensure that the seat base is level. A sling seat actively promotes adduction of the lower extremities. For a level seat base, see pages 50 (Pelvis, Level Base of Support) and 54 (Pelvis, Drop Seat Base). Measure for appropriate seat depth. If a deeper seat is required, see page 58 (Pelvis, Long Seat Base). Check for correct footrest height. Footrests that are too high will cause the lower extremities to fall either into abduction or adduction. When the client is feeling uncomfortable and unsteady sitting up in the wheelchair, an increase in the muscle tone of the lower extremities is generated. This can be due to factors such as sore buttocks or short footrests which fail to provide stability. Lastly, a positioning cushion such as the original Jay cushion can be tried, see page 45 (Pelvis, Jay Cushions). The contoured foam base has sculptured leg channels with a small abductor pommel. An abductor built-up can be added for more leg separation.

The knee abductor is always positioned between the knees and not between the thighs so that adduction is not encouraged by stimulation of the medial aspect of the thighs (Figure 5-60).

Assembly:

Medium density foam is recommended without the addition of any solid material. This is to minimize the risk of developing a pressure sore on the medial aspect of the knees after prolonged use.

The foam is cut and is rolled into a cylinder 20 cm (8 in.) long and 15 cm (6 in.) or more in diameter, big enough to maintain the legs in a neutral position.

A soft and washable fabric is used to cover the knee abductor.

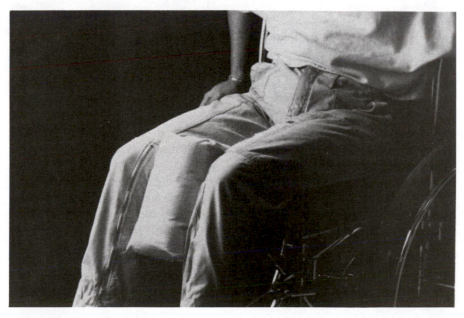

Figure 5-60. Knee abductor.

Trunk

Good trunk alignment is essential for head and neck control. Hand-eye coordination, communication, and participation in day-to-day activities such as meal management will be affected. Poor trunk alignment is likely to cause stress in various areas of the body and decrease sitting tolerance.

The trunk must be balanced centrally over the pelvis, the base of support. Stability and integrity of the spinal curvature depend on the integrity of the vertebrae, the position of the pelvis, and good muscular support. Physical changes, such as scoliosis, will change the center of gravity and the ability to balance the trunk over the pelvis. The natural tendency of the thoracic spine is to collapse forward with the effect of gravity. The able-bodied person compensates for this in sitting by crossing the arms on the chest, which slightly extends the thoracic spine, or by crossing the legs, which rotates the pelvis forward, thus increasing the lumbar lordosis which increases the extension of the thoracic spine. The disabled client, unable to compensate for the thoracic kyphosis, tends to slide down in the wheelchair to provide that stability and to maintain the head in an upright position. If the lower parts of the body, i.e., feet, legs, pelvis, and trunk, are stable, the upper body, i.e., trunk, head and upper extremities, are free for activity.

Good back support prevents or minimizes back pain and improves comfort, especially for clients with conditions such as scoliosis or osteoporosis where the integrity of the spine is destroyed. Sitting tolerance increases as pain decreases, and improvement in feelings of well-being are likely. The need for pain medication may be decreased or alleviated.

The back supports described are not intended to correct spinal deformities, but rather to accommodate them in order to improve comfort and sitting tolerance.

Potential Problems

Leaning
When sitting in the wheelchair, the client leans to one side, forward, or backward.
- This may be caused by slight to severe hypertonicity of certain muscle groups in the trunk which can affect one or both sides.
- Increased extensor tone in the trunk and extensor spasm can cause the client to push backward. This is often increased or stimulated by sitting in a wheelchair with a backrest that is too low for the client. When the backrest ends below the scapulae providing support to the lower back, it leaves the upper trunk free to go into extension. A problem of sliding forward and out of the wheelchair is often the result of this difficulty.
- Hypertonicity of various muscle groups of the trunk can also cause leaning. One or both sides may be affected to a varying degree and range from minimal to severe involvement.
- Weakness may also result in leaning.
- Leaning is often related to fatigue. It should be determined whether the client

always leans to the same side and how long he or she has been up in the wheelchair when this occurs.

Constant leaning can be the result of or can lead to fixed postural deformities such as kyphosis and scoliosis.

- Kyphosis starts with a posterior pelvic tilt, flattening or rounding out of the lumbar spine, increased thoracic kyphosis which leaves the mid-thorax supported against the backrest, exposed spinal processes of the thoracic spine, hyperextension of the cervical spine in an attempt to maintain the head in an upright position, or when muscles are too weak the head falls forward.
- Scoliosis starts with a combination of pelvic rotation and obliquity, lateral curvature of the spine, and rotation of lumbar and thoracic vertebrae. As the scoliosis causes the body to lean, the neck can go into exaggerated lateral flexion, rotation, and hyperextension in an attempt to keep the head in a vertical plane. If there is limited muscle strength, the head may follow the side of the lean.

Pain

The inability to maintain the normal curvatures of the spine results in poor alignment of the vertebrae. Pain is caused by the elevated intradiscal pressure and uneven loading of invertebral discs, ligaments, and muscles. Bending of the trunk is thought to be a contributing factor in compression fractures of the spinal vertebrae.

Back pain and poor sitting tolerance may also be due to conditions such as osteoarthritis or osteoporosis with or without compression fractures of vertebrae.

When assessing the client, note any position that provides relief from pain, the part of the back in which pain occurs, and sitting tolerance.

Pressure Sores

Pressure sores may occur over prominent spinal processes. In the case of severe kyphosis, they often occur over thoracic vertebrae.

Respiratory Problems

Poor trunk alignment and leaning can result in respiratory problems due to the limited ability to expand the lungs fully and impairment of cough.

Special Considerations

- A level and stable base is required prior to positioning the trunk. Consideration should be given first to the pelvis and second to the lower extremities as the pelvis provides the foundation and well-supported lower extremities contribute stability. This is always a priority as, for example, a scoliotic posture may be the result of pelvic obliquity. With a level and stable base enhancing the body's natural ability to maintain the upright posture, positioning intervention may be unnecessary. For further details, see Chapter 2 (Basic Sitting Position in a Wheelchair).
- A wheelchair that is too wide will be unsupportive and promote leaning. The buttocks slide to one side and the client then leans to the other side. One solution is to change the wheelchair for one of an appropriate size; see Chapter 2 (Basic Sitting Position in a Wheelchair).

- When there is no alternative to using a wheelchair that is too wide it may be difficult to mobilize the wheelchair using the upper extremities.
- The addition of a back cushion to a wheelchair without removing the sling back decreases the seat depth. According to the thickness of the cushion provided, the client may feel insecure as body weight is moved forward. This results in increased pressure over the buttocks as less support is provided for the thighs, increased difficulty mobilizing the wheelchair as the rear wheels are then situated behind the client, and increased rolling resistance as some of the body weight is moved over the front casters. In some cases, the wheelchair may tend to tip forward with the change in weight distribution.
- Increasing the height of the back may impede mobilization of the wheelchair with the upper extremities.
- When deciding on the most appropriate type of trunk support, consideration should be given to the client's ability to transfer into the wheelchair and the ability to mobilize the wheelchair.

Possible Solutions
- Foam side cushion
- Hook-on headrest (Everest and Jennings)
- Semi-reclining or fully reclining wheelchair
- Tilt-in-space wheelchair
- Padded chest restraint
    Padded chest restraint
    Padded chest restraint with shoulder straps
- Otto Bock sternal support (Otto Bock)
- Posey "Y" wheelchair safety belt (J.T. Posey)
- Otto Bock spherical side thoracic support (Otto Bock)
- Lateral support with padded armrest
- Padded lateral support
- Back cushion
- Lumbar backrest cushion
    Lumbar backrest foam cushion
    Jay combi contoured lumbar support (Jay Medical Ltd)
- Soft T-foam back cushion
- Firm contour back supports
    Jay Active back (Jay Medical Ltd)
    KSS back (Special Health Systems)
    QA2 seat back with thoracic support (QA2 Seating System)
    Jay back (Jay Medical Ltd)
    Jay Care back (Jay Medical Ltd)
    Avanti Personal back (Invacare Corp)
- Jay Modular back (Jay Medical Ltd)

Foam Side Cushion
When there is no alternative to using a wheelchair that is too wide, the addition of

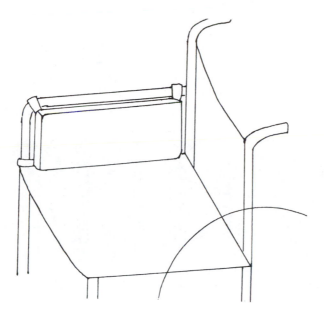

Figure 5-61. Side cushion.

side cushions (Figure 5-61) provides stability by maintaining the pelvis in a centered position.

Construction:
1. To determine the necessary thickness of the side cushions, measure across the widest part of the hips or thighs when the client is seated. Add 2.5 cm (1 in.).
2. Subtract the width of the wheelchair seat from this measurement. Include in the seat measurement, the width of the space between the side edge of the seat canvas and the armrest's side panel.
3. Divide by two to determine the thickness of each side cushion.
4. Measure the length and height inside the armrest to determine the length and width of the cushion.
5. Medium density foam is preferable.
6. Cover the cushions with any type of fabric. Use leatherette when waterproofing is necessary.
7. Sew a length of webbing or Velcro to the upper corners of each cover to attach the side cushion to the armrest.

Hook-On Headrest (Everest and Jennings)

For mild problems of trunk control, the hook-on headrest will provide trunk stability; prevent hyperextension of the upper trunk, head, and neck; and provide upper trunk support for tall clients.

This type of support does not prevent the client from leaning forward or to the side. The hook-on headrest is used in conjunction with a standard adult wheelchair.

Assembly:

The metal supports of the hook-on headrest are easily attached to the back posts of a standard adult wheelchair (Figures 5-62A and 62B).

The leatherette cover is available in two standard sizes: 41 and 46 cm (16 and 18 in.) wide. It adds 33 cm (13 in.) to the back height of the wheelchair.

If you wish to make your own cover use a strong fabric such as leather or leatherette.

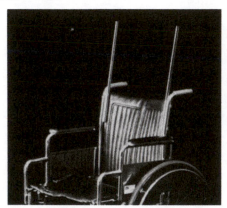 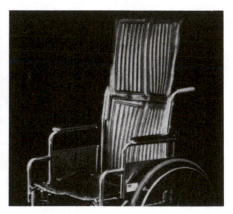

Figures 5-62A and 62B. Hook-on headrest.

Semi-Reclining or Fully Reclining Wheelchair

For the client who leans forward or to the side when using a standard wheelchair, where the leaning increases with fatigue, a reclining wheelchair can be the first step in providing increased trunk support and improving trunk alignment. By reclining the back of the wheelchair, some of the effects of gravity on the spine are eliminated. The force of gravity is spread more evenly along the spine, buttocks, and thighs and no longer applies directly down through the spine as when held in a vertical position (Figure 5-63). Therefore, less muscle work is required to maintain the spine in an upright position. A reclining wheelchair can also be used to alleviate severe back pain.

It is important not to exceed 100 degrees of hip extension in a reclining wheelchair to prevent a posterior pelvic tilt, sliding forward, and skin breakdown from the shearing forces. The use of a ramp foam cushion or wedge cushion is effective for this purpose. Be aware that the use of ramp and wedge cushions increases the seat height at the front which may make standing transfers hazardous and create environmental difficulties such as getting the knees under a table. Footrests may become too low even at their highest position. Check for correct armrest height. The use of adjustable height armrests is advisable for good trunk support. Additional positioning adaptations may be necessary after reassessment of the client in the reclining wheelchair.

Tilt-in-Space Wheelchair

The tilt-in-space wheelchair is used for the same reasons as the semi-reclining or fully reclining wheelchair. It provides trunk control and improves alignment of the spine. The tilt-in-space wheelchair can be used to alleviate back pain (see Figure 5-63).

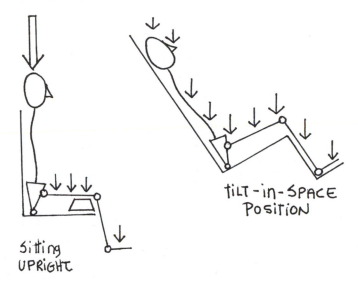

Figure 5-63. Effects of gravity on the spine.

The tilt-in-space wheelchair has the added advantage that it can be tilted in space without changing the seat to footrest and seat to back angle. It eliminates the need to use wedge cushions to maintain the hip at 100 degrees.

Depending on the client's level of functioning, the angle of tilt can be varied to provide a more upright working position and a position of rest. Standing transfer is made possible by setting the tilt-in-space wheelchair in an upright position.

Additional positioning adaptations may be necessary after reassessment of the client sitting in the tilt-in-space wheelchair.

Padded Chest Restraint

The padded chest restraint is a large foam pad placed over the chest and tied at the back of the wheelchair preventing leaning forward (Figure 5-64). It is effective in correcting mild problems of poor trunk posture related to fatigue or due to generalized increased tone in the trunk muscles.

This chest restraint does not prevent the client from leaning to the side. If required, padded shoulder straps can be added to the chest restraint to provide extra support to the upper trunk.

Padded Chest Restraint
Construction:
1. Use 2.5 cm (1 in.) low density foam.
2. To determine the length of foam required, with the client sitting in the wheelchair measure across the chest from one back post to the other. The strip of foam should be about 14 cm (5.5 in.) wide.
3. The foam is covered with 16 cm (6.5 in.) wide stockinette or any soft fabric.

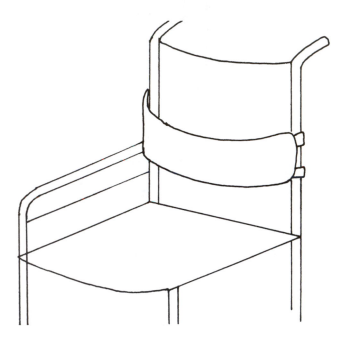

Figure 5-64. Padded chest restraint.

4. Four lengths of Velcro are sewn, one on each corner, to attach the padded chest restraint to the wheelchair.

Padded Chest Restraint With Shoulder Straps
Construction:
1. Use 2.5 cm (1 in.) low density foam and 5 cm (2 in.) wide stockinette.
2. Cut two lengths of foam 5 cm (2 in.) wide and 46 cm (18 in.) long.
3. Cut two lengths of stockinette 70 cm (28 in.) long.
4. The two lengths of foam are covered with stockinette.
5. The shoulder straps are sewn on the top and in the middle of the padded chest restraint 6 cm (2.5 in.) apart.
6. Velcro is sewn on the other end of the shoulder strap to attach it to the wheelchair push handles.
7. The shoulder straps cross at the back behind the neck (Figure 5-65).

Otto Bock Sternal Support (Otto Bock)
The Otto Bock sternal support (Figure 5-66) is an "X"-shaped polyurethane foam pad that is placed over the sternum. The two top parts of the "X" fit halfway between the neck and shoulders. The two bottom parts of the "X" are in line with the thighs. It is fixed to the wheelchair with four quick release buckles or Velcro straps. It is effective

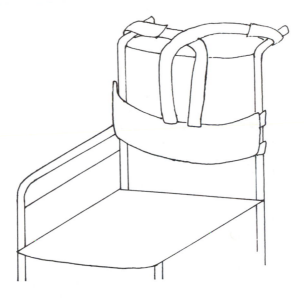

Figure 5-65. Padded chest restraint with shoulder straps.

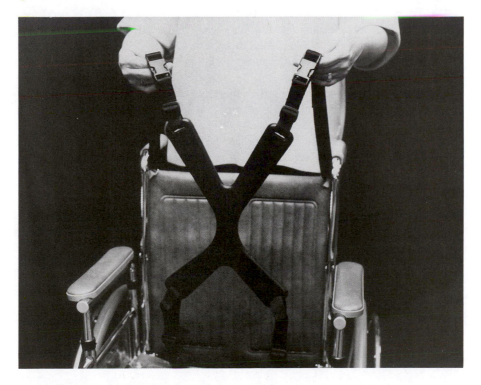

Figure 5-66. Otto Bock sternal support.

in preventing forward leaning related to fatigue or due to generalized increased tone in the trunk muscles. If leaning is due to hypotonicity or muscle weakness, it is recommended to first consider the use of a reclining wheelchair or tilt-in-space wheelchair to alleviate the effect of gravity on the spine. See page 88 (Trunk, Semi-Reclining or Fully Reclining Wheelchair and Tilt-in-Space Wheelchair).

The Otto Bock sternal support does not prevent the client from leaning to the side.

Assembly:

The sternal support pad is available in two adult sizes: intermediate and large. The overall width and height of the intermediate pad is 16.5 x 24 cm (6.5 x 9.5 in.). The large pad is 24 x 36 cm (9.5 x 14.25 in.).

To measure for the sternal support pad size:

• Width: measure 7.5 cm (3 in.) from the lateral aspect of one shoulder to 7.5 cm (3 in.) from the other shoulder. The straps will then fit halfway between the neck and shoulders without rubbing on the neck or sliding off the shoulder.

• Height: with the client sitting, measure 7.5 cm (3 in.) from the top of the shoulder to 7.5 cm (3 in.) from the top of the thighs.

The sternal support is fixed to the top screw and the bottom screw of each back post with four quick release Velcro or buckle straps. When adjusting the straps, ensure that they are not so tight as to pull downward on the shoulders.

Posey "Y" Wheelchair Safety Belt (J.T. Posey)

The Posey "Y" wheelchair safety belt (Figures 5-67A and 67B) is used as a reminder to discourage leaning forward. This safety belt is effective with clients who lean forward but who are able to correct their position.

It is ineffective when leaning is caused by fatigue and trunk weakness and also will not prevent side leaning.

It comes in one adult size but is easily adjustable to most sizes and fits most types of wheelchairs. The "Y" belt is made of strong, washable webbing.

Assembly:

The two top straps of the "Y" belt go over the shoulders and attach to the wheelchair push handles. A second long belt runs through a hole in the bottom of the "Y" belt and crosses at the back of the wheelchair attaching to the kick spurs. It is easy to put on or remove.

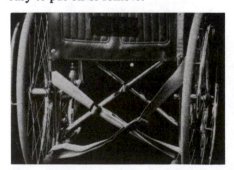 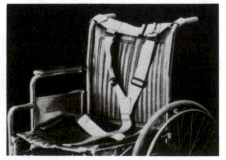

Figures 5-67A and 67B. Posey "Y" wheelchair safety belt.

Otto Bock Spherical Side Thoracic Support (Otto Bock)

This thoracic support prevents leaning to one side especially when leaning is due to hypertonicity of the trunk muscles. This support may slow the progression of a scoliosis or correct a mild one.

It is not recommended for the client who uses a standard wheelchair and is leaning due to fatigue or due to weakness of the trunk muscles. It will not prevent the client from leaning forward. See page 88 (Trunk, Semi-Reclining or Fully Reclining Wheelchair and Tilt-in-Space Wheelchair).

The use of this support will not affect the method of transfer because the support pad can be raised and swung to the side. When supporting the client it locks in place. Movement of the upper extremities is not impeded by the support.

Assembly:

The spherical thoracic supports can be fitted to the back post or armrest of any type of wheelchair. They are fully and easily adjustable to accommodate any body build.

The support pads are available in three sizes: small, medium, and large. The three styles of rod assembly—regular, extended, and dropped—are adapted specifically for right or left sides. Various sizes of mounting hardware are available to accommodate different sizes of back post. The thoracic supports can be used singly or as a pair depending on the client's needs.

The large support pad with the regular rod assembly is the most commonly used combination (Figures 5-68A and 68B). When fitting a client with the Otto Bock thoracic support, check that it is not positioned too high causing pressure on the axilla.

Lateral Support With Padded Armrest

This lateral support is used when leaning to the side is due to hypertonicity of muscles of the trunk. It is also effective in preventing mild to moderate slumping to the side due to weakness of trunk muscles. The leaning may be related to fatigue.

It provides good support to the upper extremity but does not permit functional use of the arm. It does not prevent leaning forward.

The lateral support with padded armrest can be fitted on standard adult, semi-reclining, and fully reclining wheelchairs.

Construction:

1. Use 1 cm (3/8 in.) plywood.

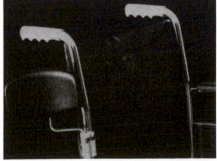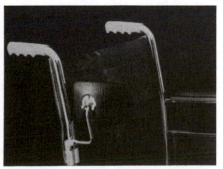

Figures 5-68A and 68B. Otto Bock spherical side thoracic support with large size support pad and right regular rod assembly.

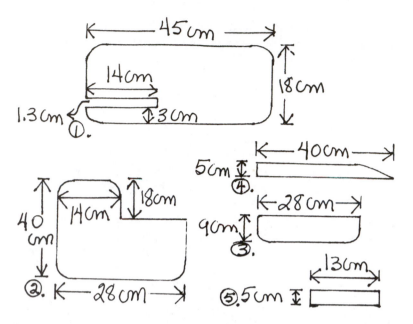

Figure 5-69. Diagram of lateral support.

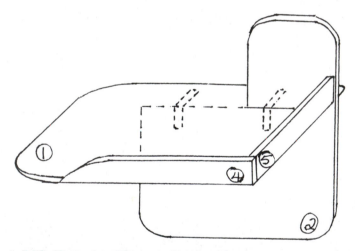

Figure 5-70. Pieces 4 and 5 secured to piece 1.

2. Cut the following pieces as shown in Figure 5-69.
3. Piece 2 fits in the slot in the piece 1. They are fixed together with two 3 cm (1.25 in.) corner braces and screws.
4. Pieces 4 and 5 are fixed to piece 1 with screws and glue (Figure 5-70).
5. Piece 3 is fixed to piece 1 with two corner braces and screws (Figure 5-71). Piece 3 is 5.5 cm (2.25 in.) from piece 2.
6. The lateral support with armrest is padded with 2.5 cm (1 in.) low density foam. The foam is stapled to the lateral support with armrest (Figure 5-72).

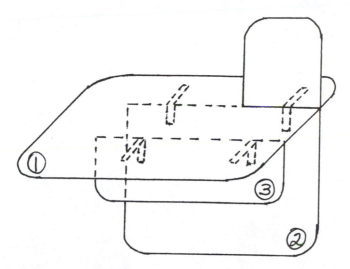

Figure 5-71. Piece 3 secured to piece 1.

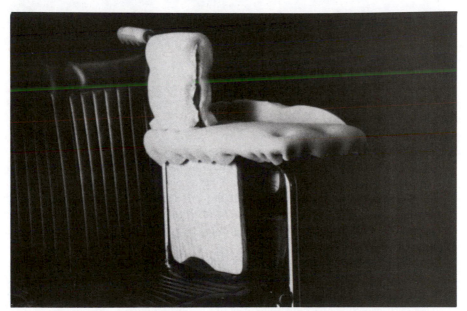

Figure 5-72. Foam padded lateral support with armrest.

7. The lateral support with padded armrest can be covered with any durable fabric such as denim. The cover is stapled to the lateral support with armrest (Figure 5-73).

Padded Lateral Support

If the client leans to the side from fatigue the padded lateral support is recommended. This type of support is not intended for clients who are able to mobilize the wheelchair with their upper extremities, although the use of the upper extremities for table activities

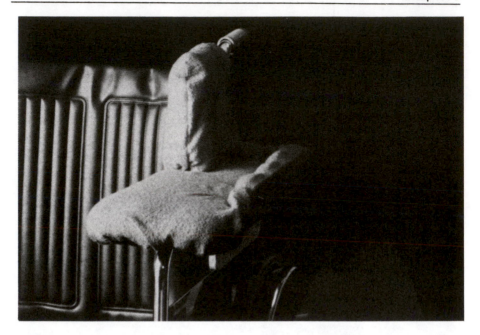

Figure 5-73. Lateral support with padded armrest.

will not be limited. Vision to the side may be restricted.

The lateral support may be used singly or as a pair and can be fitted to most types of adult wheelchair.

Construction:
1. Use 1 cm (3/8 in.) plywood.
2. Cut the following pieces as shown in Figure 5-74.
3. Piece 1 has a slight angle to accommodate the angle on the back post of the standard adult wheelchair. To determine the angle draw a line on cardboard along the back post from the rear handle to the armrest (the pad is removed) with the base of the cardboard resting on the armrest. The reclining wheelchair does not have any angle to the back post.
4. Pieces 1, 2, and 3 are fixed together with two 5 cm (2 in.) long bolts. The nuts are on the outside of the support.
5. A 3 cm (1.25 in.) corner brace is bolted so it lines up with a screw situated on the back post leaving a space the thickness of the post (Figure 5-75).
6. The lateral support is padded with 2.5 cm (1 in.) low density foam. Cover with any durable fabric such as denim. The cover is stapled to the lateral support.
7. The padded lateral support (Figure 5-76) sits on the armrest and is fixed to the back post using the screw from the back upholstery and the corner brace.
8. Pieces 2 (see Figure 5-74) should be longer if the lateral support is fitted to a reclining wheelchair.

Back Cushion
The purpose of a back cushion is to improve comfort. Sitting tolerance may

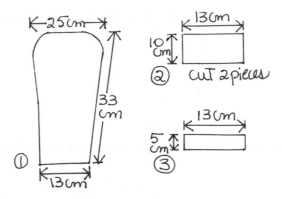

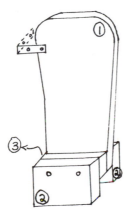

Figure 5-74. Diagram of padded lateral support.

Figure 5-75. Right lateral support.

increase as back pain is controlled.

A back cushion may be an effective solution for clients who complain of back pain but do not suffer from spinal deformities that would require additional support.

There is no certain way to determine which type of cushion is most appropriate. Personal preference for a soft or firm cushion may be indicated by the client. The most appropriate type of cushion will be determined by trial and error.

Back cushions can be fitted to any type of wheelchair and should be secured, usually to the back frame, to prevent slipping (Figure 5-77).

Construction:

1. Use 2.5 cm (1 in.) low or medium density foam depending on how firm a cushion is required. Eggcrate foam 2.5 cm (1 in.) low density can be used for a soft back cushion.
2. The cushion is cut to the size of the wheelchair's back upholstery.
3. A soft and stretchy fabric is used to cover the foam cushion.

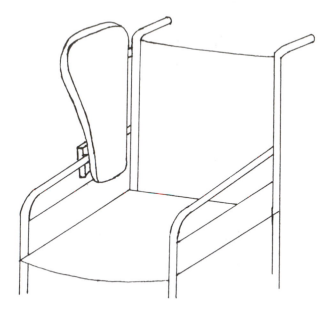

Figure 5-76. Padded lateral support.

4. Two lengths of webbing are sewn to the upper corners to attach the back cushion
   to the rear handles of the wheelchair.

Lumbar Backrest Cushion

This cushion provides support to the lumbar region. It assists in restoring the
natural lumbar curve thus promoting improved posture in the thoracic and cervical
spine. It helps to reduce fatigue and decrease back pain.

The lumbar cushion can be fitted on any type of wheelchair. Using a lumbar
backrest cushion with clients who have increased extensor tone in the trunk and hips,
tight hamstrings, poor hip flexion, or marked kyphotic posture is not recommended.
These clients are unable to tilt their pelvis forward to achieve a lumbar lordosis. The
pelvis can be fixed in a posterior tilt. The lumbar cushion may increase extensor tone
and the tendency to slide forward in the wheelchair.

Lumbar Backrest Foam Cushion
Construction:
1. Use 2.5 or 5 cm (1 or 2 in.) low density foam depending on the client's need.
   Eggcrate foam can also be used.
2. It is usually 20 cm (8 in.) high and is cut to fit the width of the wheelchair.
3. It is covered with stockinette or any soft and stretchy fabric.
4. Four lengths of Velcro are sewn one in each corner to attach the cushion to the
   wheelchair (Figure 5-78).

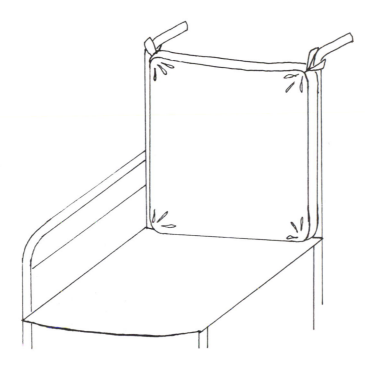

Figure 5-77. Foam back cushion.

Jay Combi Contoured Lumbar Support (Jay Medical Ltd)
Assembly:
The combi contoured lumbar support (Figure 5-79) is made of low density foam and has a removable foam insert for custom fitting. It is secured to the wheelchair push handles with two Velcro straps.

Soft T-Foam Back Cushion
This back cushion is made of soft T-foam which molds to accommodate bony prominences of the spine and is especially useful for emaciated clients. It helps prevent pressure sores and improves sitting comfort.
Construction:
1. Use 1.3 or 2.5 cm (0.5 or 1 in.) soft T-foam. It is usually cut to fit the size of the back of the wheelchair.
2. The cushion can be covered with any soft and stretchy fabric. It is attached to the wheelchair with ties which are sewn in the upper corners of the cover.

Firm Contour Back Supports
As the back canvas stretches, the pelvis falls into a posterior tilt. This in turn induces a flattening of the lumbar spine or lumbar kyphosis. The absence of a normal

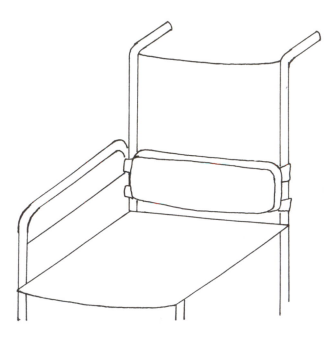

Figure 5-78. Lumbar backrest foam cushion.

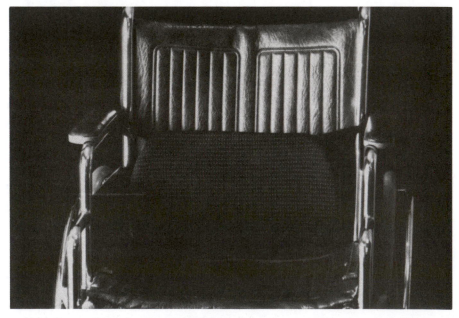

Figure 5-79. Jay combi contoured backrest.

lumbar lordosis affects the integrity of the spine with an increase in thoracic kyphosis and hyperextension of the cervical spine in an effort to maintain the head in an upright position (see Figure 5-3). Concurrently, the tendency to slide forward and out of the wheelchair is increased. For clients with conditions such as osteoporosis, osteoarthritis, and compression fractures of the vertebrae, the hammock effect of the wheelchair's sling back can contribute to an increase in back pain and poor sitting tolerance.

A rigid back support assists in promoting good alignment of the spine by providing firm support to the pelvis and trunk. Thus back pain can be decreased and sitting tolerance improved.

Except for the Jay Active back, the firm contour back supports described can be fitted with lateral supports for further positioning of the trunk.

A firm back support should not be given to a client without also providing a firm seat base in order to maintain a level pelvis.

Jay Active Back (Jay Medical Ltd)

The Jay Active back is used to provide comfortable upright sitting. It helps to restore and maintain the normal curvatures of the spine. It is not designed for clients who are at risk for leaning or who have a fixed postural deformity.

There are two types of back cushion: the Jay Active back and the tall Jay Active back (Figure 5-80). The tall Jay Active back is intended for taller clients or clients who need more support from the back.

The Jay Active backs can be fitted to most types of standard adult wheelchair with

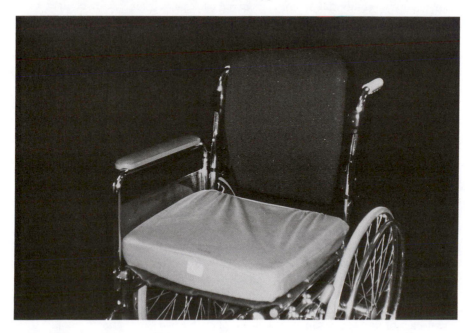

Figure 5-80. Tall Jay Active back.

widths ranging from 36 to 46 cm (14 to 18 in.). The length of the Jay Active back is 31 cm (12 in.) with height adjustment from 31 to 41 cm (12 to 16 in.). The length of the tall Jay Active back is 41 cm (16 in.) with height adjustment from 36 to 46 cm (14 to 18 in.).

The Jay Active back has a rigid back shell with a contoured foam support and an air-exchange cover.

Assembly:

With the sling back removed, it is fitted on the back posts with two quick-release brackets. Elevating or lowering the brackets provide height adjustment. The quick-release mechanism permits installation and removal of the back for folding and transportation of the wheelchair. Additional adjustments to customize the Jay Active backs include a back angle wedge for more vertical sitting and an adjustable lumbar support pad. They are fitted between the back shell and the foam support with Velcro.

KSS Back (Special Health Systems)

The KSS back is used to provide comfortable upright sitting. Firm support is provided to the upper body while use of the upper extremities is unrestricted. Lateral supports are options for controlling moderate problems of leaning to the side due to poor trunk control. They may assist in slowing the progression of a scoliosis or in correcting a mild one.

KSS backs are available in planar or curved models with an optional pneumatic lumbar support. The planar back is composed of a rigid base covered with 2.5 cm (1 in.) medium firm foam (Figure 5-81). The curved back is also made of a rigid curved base padded with contouring foam. The curved back provides increased contact with the client's back increasing support to the trunk. It incorporates a sacral pad that applies support on the posterior superior iliac spine. This assists in promoting a neutral pelvic position. The use of a sacral pad should be assessed carefully as it can actually increase the tone with clients who have high extensor tone in the trunk. The curved back is available with a pneumatic lumbar-thoracic adjustable support which is inflated/deflated to increase support throughout the back. KSS backs have a removable neoprene spandex cover. Standard sizes fit 41 and 46 cm (16 and 18 in.) width wheelchairs. Standard height is 50 cm (20 in.).

The lateral supports can be fixed or swing-away (see Figure 5-81). The swing-away bracket permits easier transfer into the wheelchair and prevents injury to the back when getting in the wheelchair. When the support is slightly lifted the pad will swing to the side. The lateral support swings back and locks into place as the client sits back into the wheelchair. The pads are covered with medium density foam or contouring foam, and removable Coolmax covers. Standard pad size is 14 cm (5.5 in.) height by 21.5 cm (8.5 in.) depth. The lateral supports are ordered singly. It is necessary to specify right or left and planar or curved back.

Custom sizes are available for all KSS backs and lateral supports.

Assembly:

With the sling back removed, the KSS back is suspended in a slight recline on the vertical bars of the wheelchair. It is held in place by two "anti-gravity hooks" that also permit back height adjustment. The KSS backs can be easily lifted and removed for folding and transportation of the wheelchair. The lateral supports attach to the

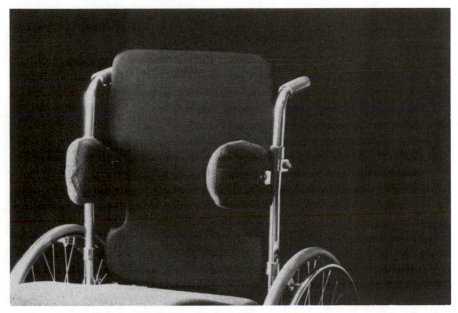

Figure 5-81. KSS planar back with lateral supports.

KSS back with a steel bracket. They are adjustable in width in 1.25 cm (0.5 in.) increments. Height adjustment is accomplished by elevating or lowering the KSS back's brackets on the back posts.

QA2 Seat Back With Thoracic Support (QA2 Seating System)

The QA2 seat back with thoracic supports is used to provide firm support to the trunk and promote good alignment of the spine (Figure 5-82).

It can also be used with clients who are at risk for side leaning or who are leaning slightly to the side due to poor trunk control. For more effective prevention of leaning, this system is used in conjunction with a reclining wheelchair.

The QA2 seat back with thoracic support can be fitted to most types of standard adult and reclining wheelchairs with widths ranging from 36 to 51 cm (14 to 20 in.).

Assembly:

The QA2 seat back is used with the regular or drop seat base; see pages 52 (Pelvis, QA2 Seat Base) and 54 (Pelvis, Drop Seat Base). The QA2 seating system is made of strong ABS thermal plastic.

Trunk support is provided and custom fitting is possible as the two thoracic supports are attached to the seat back with dual-lock (a type of industrial Velcro).

With the sling seat removed the seating system inserts into the wheelchair. A strap secures the seat back to the wheelchair.

Jay Back (Jay Medical Ltd)

The Jay back is an adjustable wheelchair back (Figure 5-83). It provides trunk

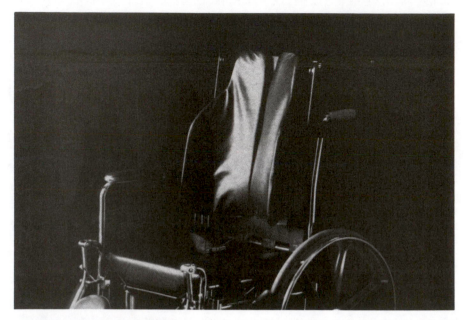

Figure 5-82. QA2 seating system.

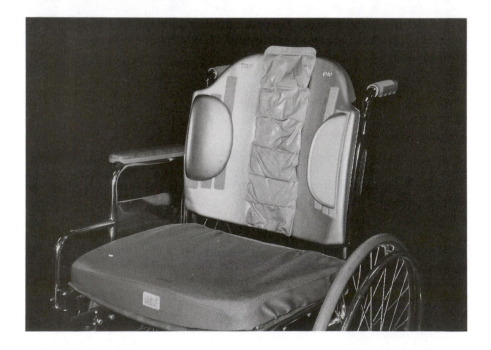

Figure 5-83. Jay back.

stability and can help control back pain. It can be easily customized to provide support and comfort for clients with mild kyphosis and scoliosis. The flolite spinal insert is a fluid pad which reduces pressure on bony protusions of the spine and helps to prevent skin breakdown.

The tall Jay back (Figure 5-84) is 12.5 cm (5 in.) taller providing 15 cm (6 in.) of support above the scapula. A scapular recess allows good mobility at the shoulder for easy wheeling. Intended for tall clients, the tall Jay back can be used for shorter clients who need extra support or on reclining wheelchairs. The tall Jay back can also be effective in positioning clients with increased extensor tone by providing full support to the trunk. The Jay back can be fitted to most types of standard adult and reclining wheelchairs with widths ranging from 33 to 51 cm (13 to 20 in.). Height adjustment ranges from 33 to 56 cm (13 to 22 in.).

The tall Jay back can be fitted to most types of standard adult and reclining wheelchairs with widths ranging from 38 to 46 cm (15 to 18 in.). Height adjustment ranges from 43 to 68 cm (17 to 27 in.).

The Jay back has a rigid back shell with contoured foam support, a flolite spinal insert, and an air-exchange cover.

Accessories to customize the Jay back include a back wedge for more vertical sitting, an adjustable lumbar support pad, and two adjustable lateral foam supports. The lateral supports are adjustable independently in height, width, and rotation. Extra-large lateral supports are available. The lateral supports are effective with clients who are at risk for side leaning or who are leaning slightly to the side due to poor trunk control. The accessories are fitted to the contoured foam back support with Velcro.

Assembly:

With the sling back removed, the Jay back is fitted to the back posts with two brackets. Elevating or lowering the brackets provide height adjustment. The Jay back

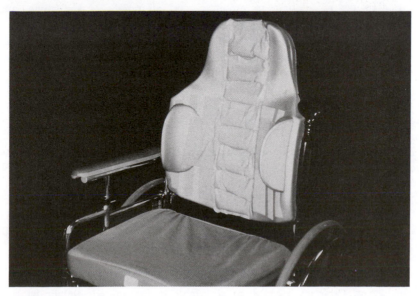

Figure 5-84. Tall Jay back.

is fixed to the bracket with a twist lock latch and can be easily removed for folding and transportation of the wheelchair.

Jay Care Back (Jay Medical Ltd)

Jay Care back (see Figure 5-16) is an anatomically designed contoured back support which provides pressure relief along the spine and accommodates a mild to moderate kyphotic posture. A regular wheelchair's sling seat and back promote a posterior pelvic tilt and sacral sitting, or rounding out of the lower spine, which is accompanied by an increased thoracic kyphosis. The cervical spine is often hyperextended trying to maintain the head in an upright position or the head drops forward when strength and mobility are limited (see Figure 5-3). This type of kyphotic posture is often encountered within the older adult population who spend numerous hours each day sitting in a wheelchair. The Jay Care back helps control the progression of a kyphosis, decreases back pain, and promotes a more comfortable upright sitting posture.

The Jay Care back is made of an ABS plastic structural shell and soft foam. The plastic structural shell has built-in lateral supports. The soft foam has a segmental central section to increase conformity to bony prominences of the spine and to prevent skin breakdown. The Jay Care back is adjustable in height, angle, and depth. The mounting hardware allows the Jay Care back to be easily removed from the wheelchair for transportation. The Jay Care back cover is made of washable stretch material.

The Jay Care back is intended to be used primarily in conjunction with the Jay Care cushion to create the Jay Care seating system; see page 49 (Pelvis, Jay Care Cushion) for additional information. It helps solve common seating problems resulting from the wheelchair sling seat and back. The Jay Care seating system is designed to position the pelvis and the lower extremities, to prevent sliding forward and out of the wheelchair, to promote good alignment of the spine, and to accommodate a mild to moderate kyphotic posture.

The Jay Care back is available in two standard sizes: regular adult to fit wheelchairs 43 to 45 cm wide (17 to 18 in.) and narrow adult to fit wheelchairs 38 to 40 cm (15 to 16 in.). The back height is 45 cm (18 in.).

Assembly:

With the sling back removed, the Jay Care back is mounted on the back posts. The back height is adjusted by elevating or lowering the mounting brackets on the back posts.

Please note, power and reclining wheelchairs usually have a rigid bar across the backrest for strength and stability. This bar can interfere with the installation of the backrest.

Support wedges can be added to increase body contact laterally. For the client with wider hips and a narrower trunk, a 40 cm (16 in.) back can be mounted on a 45 cm (18 in.) wheelchair or a 45 cm (18 in.) back can be mounted on a 51 cm (20 in.) wheelchair. Check with a Jay representative for special ordering number.

Avanti Personal Back (Invacare Corp)

The Avanti Personal back is an adjustable contoured wheelchair back. It is designed to maintain proper alignment of the spine and to provide side-to-side trunk stability. The Avanti Personal back can also be used to position the client with a mild kyphotic posture related to sitting in a wheelchair with a sling seat and back (see Figure 5-3). Adequate support and proper alignment of the spine will often promote a more upright sitting posture, improved sitting tolerance, and decreased back pain.

The Avanti Personal back is made of an ABS thermal plastic back shell lined with a 2.5 cm (1 in.) comfort foam. The removable zip-closure cover is made of a two-way stretch material. The Avanti Personal back has a removable foam lumbar support and two lateral wedges which increase body contact and support as needed.

The Avanti Personal back is usually fitted to a standard adult wheelchair with widths ranging from 30 to 51 cm (12 to 20 in.). It is available in two standard heights: 40 and 46 cm (16 and 18 in.) or 48 cm (19 in.) tall. The Avanti Personal back tall (Figure 5-85) can be used to position tall clients or clients who need for example extra support to the trunk due to high extensor tone. The back is fitted to the wheelchair with quick-release attachment brackets for ease of transport. Three positions on the upper and lower brackets allow for back height, seat depth, and angle adjustment. By changing the locations of the top and bottom mounts, it is possible to increase the seat depth of up to 5 cm (2 in.) or to recline the backrest up to 30 degrees.

Assembly:

Please note, power and reclining wheelchairs usually have a rigid bar across the backrest for strength and stability. This bar can interfere with the installation of the backrest.

With the wheelchair sling back removed, the Avanti Personal back attachment brackets are fitted to the back posts. Height adjustment is accomplished by elevating or lowering the mounting brackets on the back posts. Three types of mounting brackets are available. The first type is fitted to the back posts with screws into

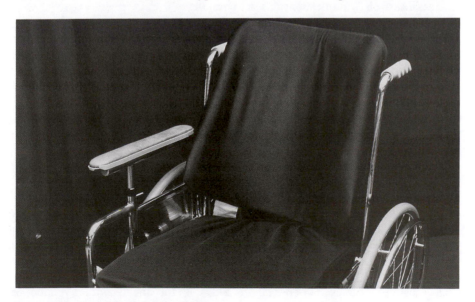

Figure 5-85. Avanti Personal back tall.

existing upholstery mount holes. There are several holes on the mounting bracket to choose from to allow for back adjustment. This type of bracket is preferable for long-term use as it will not slide on the back post over time.

The second type is mounted as securely as the first type but requires drilling of new holes in the back posts to mount the Avanti back. The therapist must determine the exact back height prior to fitting the brackets.

The third type uses clamps to attach the brackets to the back posts. It is ideal for assessment purposes but be cautious if using over the long term as it is possible that the clamps will loosen allowing the brackets to move on the back posts.

Jay Modular Back (Jay Medical Ltd)

The Jay Modular back is designed to accommodate clients with limited hip flexion, a kyphotic or moderately scoliotic spine, and clients who cannot tolerate verticality.

The Jay Modular back includes an adjustable aluminum shell which provides variable seat depth, back height, and degree of recline. Adjustment possibilities are as follow: 7.5 cm (3 in.) seat depth, 43 to 56 cm (17 to 22 in.) back height from top of seat rails to top of back shell, and 49 degrees of backward recline from vertical. The aluminum back shell is sturdy enough for a bolted-on headrest attachment. It can be fitted with two types of insert: standard or custom contoured. The Jay Modular back also includes a breathable air-exchange cover. Because of the amount of recline possible, the Jay Modular back is usually fitted on a standard adult wheelchair. It is available in widths ranging from 35 to 51 cm (14 to 20 in.).

Jay Medical offers literature on how to fit and use the Jay Modular back. It is strongly recommended that the modular back be assessed on the client by a trained therapist or dealer prior to purchase due to the variety of adjustments, combinations of accessories, and modifications that are possible.

Assembly:

Please note, power and reclining wheelchairs usually have a rigid bar across the backrest for strength and stability. This bar can interfere with the installation of the backrest.

With the sling back removed, the Jay Modular back shell suspends on the vertical bars of the wheelchair with clamp-on hardware and top quick-release brackets. Clamp-on hardware allows for easy change of height for evaluation. Screw-on hardware is optional but recommended for long-term use. The top quick release brackets lock the back in place and twist away for quick removal of the back.

When setting the back shell in a fully reclined position on a standard wheelchair, it is advisable to assess the need for anti-tippers or amputee axle adapter brackets.

The aluminum back shell is then fitted with one of the two type of inserts:

- The standard insert (Figure 5-86) is for clients without significant back deformities. It is a 7.5 cm (3 in.) thick polyethelene closed-cell foam with a 16 cm (6.5 in.) wide spinal flolite fluid pad. It is feasible to cut away foam from the standard insert and then to add a flolite pad to relieve pressure on minor bony deformities.
- The custom contoured insert (Figure 5-87) is for clients with kyphotic or moderately scoliotic spinal deformity. It is made of light polyethelene closed-cell foam. The insert is composed of a 1.5 cm (0.5 in.) thick shim and covered with 6.5

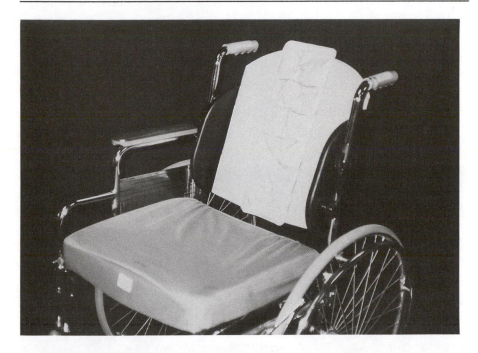

Figure 5-86. Jay Modular back with standard insert.

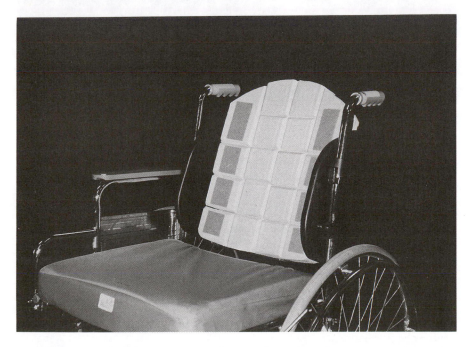

Figure 5-87. Jay Modular back with custom contoured insert.

cm (2.5 in.) thick removable blocks. To fit the Jay Modular back, remove appropriate blocks that correspond to points of protruding deformities on the client's back. This permits recessing of these deformities into the back system, increasing contact surface on the client's back and distributing pressure more evenly. Transition wedges can be added in the recesses, depending on the space available, to provide a more contoured fit. The custom contoured insert is then covered with a full-width flolite fluid pad to smooth out contours and relieve pressure points (Figure 5-88).

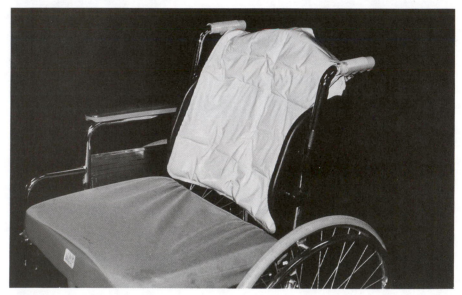

Figure 5-88. Jay Modular back with custom contoured insert and flolite pad.

To further customized the Jay Modular back, the Jay back box includes the following accessories:
- Adjustable lateral foam supports for stable side-to-side support. Available in three adult sizes.
- Extended lateral supports made of steel with foam pads. Additional wedge and flolite pad can be added for fit and pressure relief. Available in three adult sizes.
- Adjustable lumbar foam support fitted behind the flolite pad of the back insert. Available in three adult sizes.
- Transition wedges to smooth transition points when blocks are removed from the custom contoured insert. Available in corner, full, and half-width sizes.
- Two sizes of fill-in pads to build contact with deformities.
- Flolite gibbous pad to fill cut away from standard insert and to relieve pressure on a minor bony prominence.

Head and Neck

Positioning of the head and neck relies on good body alignment and support. It is directly dependent upon the position of the pelvis, alignment of the spine, and trunk stability.

The ability to maintain good head and neck position affects the performance of activities such as the time spent eating, behavior during eating, independence in eating, and the ability to keep food and liquid in the mouth. The position of the head also affects swallowing and the risk of choking. Communication with friends and family is difficult without the ability to maintain the head in an upright position in order to make eye contact. Hand-eye coordination which is needed for recreational activities such as table games also requires good head control.

Potential Problems

Poor Head Control

The head may droop forward, to one side, or fall backward.

Poor head control may result from hypertonicity, hypotonicity (slight to severe), or weakness of the muscles of the neck and can affect one side more than the other.

Spinal deformities affect the ability to maintain the head in an upright position. A kyphosis causes hyperextension of the cervical spine as the client tries to maintain the head in an upright position but if strength is limited the head will droop forward. Scoliosis results in excessive rotation and lateral flexion of the cervical spine to maintain the head upright, but when strength is limited, can cause the head to droop in the direction of the lean. Therefore, ensuring an optimal position of the pelvis and trunk is a prerequisite to the positioning of the head.

Poor head control is affected by fatigue. It should be noted whether the head always droops in the same direction and when it occurs.

Pain

The client may complain of pain in the upper back and neck. It may be related to poor head righting or conditions such as osteoarthritis or osteoporosis which affect the integrity of the vertebrae.

The assessment should note whether or not pain occurs with movement, if it is accentuated by fatigue, and if it is constantly present.

Special Considerations

- A rigid cervical collar can be effective in maintaining proper alignment of the head but it may be uncomfortable and interfere with speaking and swallowing.
- It is necessary to carefully assess the amount of support required from the headrest as the headrest can become a form of restraint. For example, a headrest which provides lateral support will restrict lateral flexion and rotation of the neck and head.
- A supportive headband attached to the wheelchair may not be acceptable to client or family for aesthetic reasons.

Possible Solutions
- Foam headrest
- Hook-on headrest (Everest and Jennings)
- Semi-reclining or fully reclining wheelchair and tilt-in-space wheelchair
- Pillow headrest
- Crown head support
  - Wooden crown head support
  - Crown head support with Otto Bock headrest attachment (Otto Bock)
- Head and neck supports—Seating systems
  - QA2 headrest (QA2 Seating System)
  - KSS neck support (Special Health Systems)
  - Otto Bock head and neck supports (Otto Bock)

Foam Headrest
When poor head control and limited strength cause the head to fall into a hyperextended position or fall to the side, the foam headrest can provide support for mild to moderate positioning problems.

This type of headrest is used in conjunction with a fully reclining or semi-reclining wheelchair with a detachable telescopic headrest.

If the head continues to droop forward when the client is positioned in a reclining wheelchair, the foam headrest will be ineffective.

Construction:
1. Use two layers of 7.5 cm (3 in.) medium density foam.
2. Two pieces of foam 24 cm (9 in.) high by 37 cm (14 in.) wide are glued together to form a block.
3. The block is carved to provide contour fitting for the head and neck following the measurements in Figure 5-89. The headrest is 9 cm (3.5 in.) thick in the middle at the bottom.
4. The measurements can be modified to fit the individual client.
5. The headrest can be covered with 17 cm (6.5 in.) wide stockinette or any soft, stretchy fabric. An elastic is sewn to the two sides of the cover to secure the headrest to the wheelchair (Figure 5-90).

Hook-On Headrest (Everest and Jennings)
The back extension is an effective support when used for problems of mild to moderate hypertonicity of the extensor muscles of the trunk and neck which causes the head to fall back.

It is also used to prevent poor head righting due to fatigue by providing support for the upper trunk, neck, and head.

Assembly:
See page 87 (Trunk, Hook-On Headrest).

Semi-Reclining or Fully Reclining Wheelchair and Tilt-in-Space Wheelchair
A reclining wheelchair with a detachable telescopic headrest or a tilt-in-space

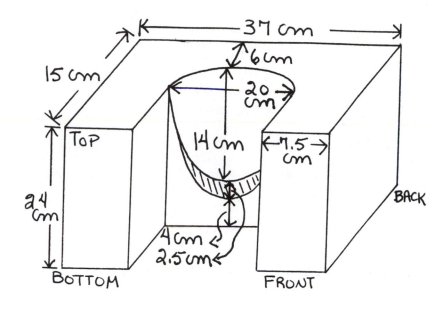

Figure 5-89. Diagram of foam headrest.

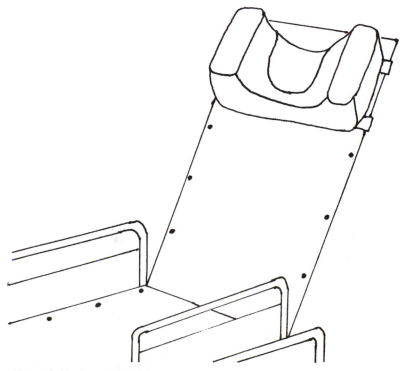

Figure 5-90. Foam headrest.

wheelchair can be an effective solution for the client whose head falls forward or to the side due to decreased tone in the extensor muscles of the neck or weakness of the muscles of the neck. The inability to maintain the head in an upright position may increase with fatigue.

The effect of gravity will hold the head back on the headrest which is used together with the reclining or tilt-in-space wheelchair.

Additional support such as a foam headrest may be needed to complete the positioning.

Pillow Headrest

A pillow headrest is recommended when minimal support will provide comfort. A pillow headrest secured to the detachable telescopic headrest of a reclining wheelchair will help to hold the head in an upright position.

Construction:

1. The open end of the pillow case is held together with Velcro so the pillow case can be easily removed and washed.
2. Two lengths of elastic 2.5 cm (1 in.) wide are sewn onto the ends of the pillow case to hold the pillow on the headrest. One length of elastic joins the upper corners and one joins the lower corners.

Crown Head Support

Clients who are unable to keep the head from drooping forward may find the crown head support useful and may learn to put it on independently when they need the extra support.

It is usually used in conjunction with a standard adult wheelchair.

Prior to fitting a crown head support, the therapist must clearly identify the cause of the problem, i.e., head drooping forward. In most cases, a head which is falling forward is the result of a kyphotic spine. Therefore, positioning of the pelvis and trunk must be addressed first.

Wooden Crown Head Support
Construction:

For a 46 cm (18 in.) wide adult wheelchair:

• Base:

1. Use 1 cm (3/8 in.) plywood for the base.
2. In the center at the top of a 20 x 48 cm (7.75 x 19 in.) board, attach a box 13 x 5 x 5 cm (5 x 2 x 2 in.) (Figure 5-91).
3. One hole is made in each corner of the board to attach it to the back of the wheelchair. These screw holes must line up with the screws on the back of the wheelchair.

• Upright support:

4. On a wooden post 56 x 2.5 x 4 cm (22 x 1 x 1.5 in.) drill three holes large enough for a 5 cm (2 in.) long bolt. They start 2.5 cm (1 in.) from the top and are 4 cm (1.5 in.) apart (Figure 5-92).

• Head band:

5. The head band is in two parts: attachment and crown.

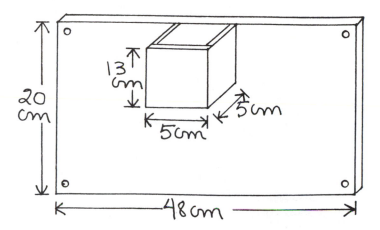

Figure 5-91. Base.

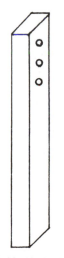

Figure 5-92. Upright support.

- Attachment:
6. Use two pieces of a low temperature thermoplastic material such as san-splint 25 x 6.5 cm (10 x 2.5 in.). Make three holes in each piece of san-splint 2.5 cm (1 in.) apart at one end and one hole at 2.5 cm (1 in.) from the other end (Figure 5-93).
- Crown:
7. One piece of 1.2 cm (0.5 in.) low temperature closed-cell foam material such as plastazote 76 x 7.5 cm (30 x 3 in.). Make one hole 4 cm (1.5 in.) from each end. The holes on the plastazote need to be reinforced with a piece 5 x 5 cm (2 x 2 in.) of any type of thin plastic. The plastazote can be covered with stockinette and

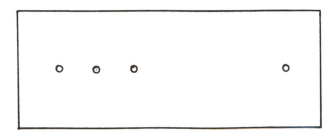

Figure 5-93. Attachment.

changed as necessary for cleanliness.
8. To assemble the head support, see Figure 5-94:
9. The board is fixed on the wheelchair.
10. The post is put in the box.
11. The two pieces of san-splint are fixed to the post with a 10 cm (4 in.) long bolt. The three holes on the post and the san-splint are for adjustments.
12. The plastazote head band is fixed to the san-splint with a 5 cm (2 in.) long bolt.
13. A 20 cm (8 in.) long piece of webbing can be sewn on the stockinette to keep the head band from falling down over the face.

Crown Head Support With Otto Bock Headrest Attachment (Otto Bock)

An alternative to the wooden crown head support is to use the wheelchair adapter kit with the headrest, multi- or single-axis, straight or offset, from Otto Bock (Figure 5-95). The wheelchair adapter kit can be fitted on any type of adult wheelchair with widths ranging from 36 to 46 cm (14 to 18 in.). The headrest hardware can be multi- or single-axis, straight or offset, depending on the amount of adjustment needed. The hardware single-axis straight or offset is adjustable in height and depth. The hardware multi-axis straight or offset provides a full range of adjustment in all three planes.

The plastazote head band described above can be easily fitted to the axis with a piece of san-splint 5 x 41 cm (2 x 16 in.) molded to fit the axis. A bolt 5 cm (2 in.) long is used to fix the head band to the piece of san-splint (see Figure 5-95).

Head and Neck Supports—Seating Systems

There are three types of fully adjustable head and neckrest supports which are part of a complete seating systems—QA2 headrest, KSS neck support, and Otto Bock head and neck supports. They are recommended for any type of positioning problem of the head or neck except when the head droops forward.

QA2 Headrest (QA2 Seating System)

The QA2 headrest is fully adjustable in height, depth, and angle. The headrest

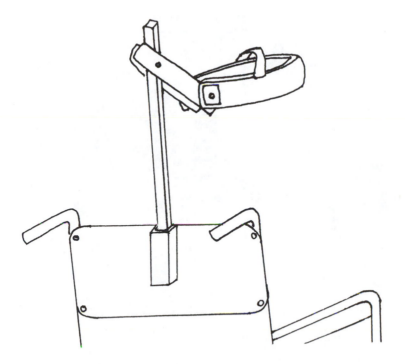

Figure 5-94. Wooden crown head support.

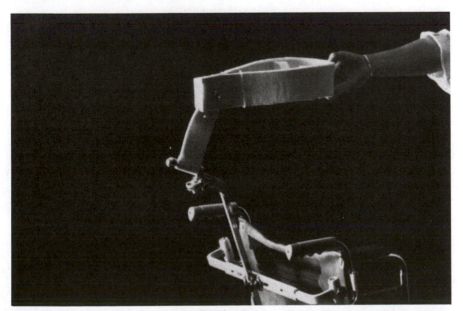

Figure 5-95. Crown head support with Otto Bock multi-axis offset headrest attachment.

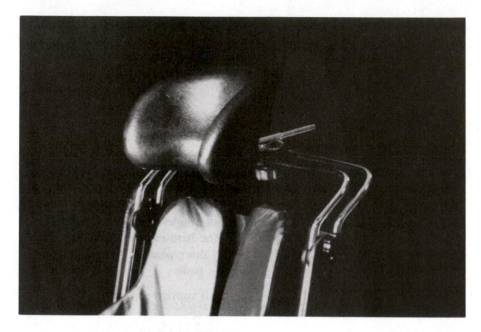

Figure 5-96. QA2 headrest with combination head and neckrest Otto Bock cushion.

hardware assembly can be fitted with any type of Otto Bock headrest cushion (Figure 5-96).

The headrest is used in conjunction with the QA2 seat and back. See page 103 (Trunk, QA2 Seat Back With Thoracic Support) for seat and back fittings.

KSS Neck Support (Special Health Systems)

The KSS neck support (Figure 5-97) is easily adjustable in height and depth. Designed to provide support to the neck and lower head it prevents hyperextension and permits lateral movement of the head.

The contoured plastic neck pad has 2.5 cm (1 in.) medium density foam padding or contour foam. The pad is available in one standard size 28 cm (11 in.) long by 10 cm (4 in.) high. It is covered with lycra and has a stretch terry cloth cover. Custom size pads are available.

The KSS neck support is used in conjunction with the KSS back. For the description and fitting of the back, see page 102 (Trunk, KSS Back).

Otto Bock Head and Neck Supports (Otto Bock)

The Otto Bock head and neck supports (Figure 5-98) can be fitted on any adult wheelchair of widths ranging from 36 to 46 cm (14 to 18 in.) using the wheelchair adapter kit.

The headrest hardware can be multi- or single-axis, straight or offset, depending on the amount of adjustment needed. The hardware single-axis straight or offset is adjustable in height and depth. The hardware multi-axis straight or offset provides

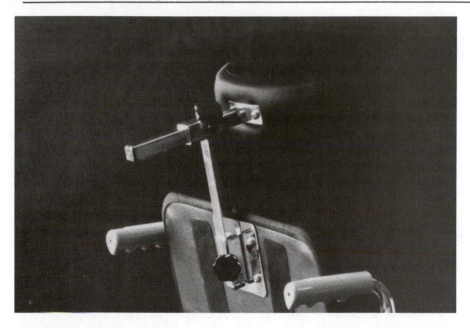

Figure 5-97. KSS neck support.

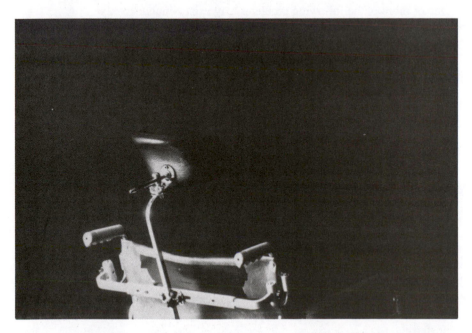

Figure 5-98. Otto Bock wheelchair adapter kit with multi-axis offset headrest hardware and combination head/neckrest support pad.

full range of adjustment in all three planes. Otto Bock offers a wide variety of support pads:

- Combination head/neckrest: Provides full support to the head and neck. It also gives lateral support.
- Neckrest (small, large, or tapered): Provides support to the neck and the lower head.
- Headrest (small and large): provides support to the head only and does not restrict lateral movement.

Upper Extremities

The prerequisite for optimal functioning of the upper extremities is a stable and symmetric sitting posture. A symmetric spine and good trunk control help in stabilizing the shoulder girdle, permitting the hands to reach and work in the body midline. Therefore, to maximize independence in activities of daily living such as self care, meal management, and mobilization of the wheelchair, positioning of the upper extremities must be preceded by an assessment of the whole sitting posture.

Intervention is necessary to position the nonfunctional upper extremity for the protection of joint integrity, muscle tone control, prevention of contractures, and alleviation of pain.

Potential Problems

One or more of the following problems may exist simultaneously:

- Subluxation of the shoulder joint. Subluxation refers to the presence of a space between the acromion process and the head of the humerus. The integrity of the joint is dependent upon muscular support. If the muscles are weak, ligaments stretch and the joint capsule is weakened resulting in subluxation of the joint. Shoulder subluxation is often accompanied by pain.
- Hypotonicity which may be slight to severe.
- Hypertonicity which may be slight to severe.
- Weakness of individual muscle groups or of the whole extremity.
- Edema which usually occurs in the hand and may extend up the wrist.
- Contractures: flexion contractures are common and may involve one or more joints.
- Perceptual deficit such as decreased awareness of an arm or visual deficit such as hemianopsia which result in the inability to see one side of the body. Fingers may get caught in the spokes of the wheel or an arm may be crushed between the wheelchair and a wall or doorway.
- Impaired sensitivity in the affected upper extremity.

Special Considerations

- The method used to transfer the client must be considered when using a wheelchair table as an aid to positioning the upper extremity as it will impede independent transferring.
- Mobility may be restricted when using a wheelchair table. Using the unaffected extremity to reach and push the hand rim will be difficult when the wheelchair

table extends past the armrests.
- The use of a wheelchair table that does not permit the client to see the lower extremities may increase perceptual problems and enhance lack of body awareness.
- It is often difficult for a client to get close to the table when using an arm trough due to its size and position on the wheelchair. The adaptation may not be acceptable for this reason. It is important to discuss with the client the necessity of the arm trough or other proposed adaptations.
- Functional use of the affected upper extremity must be carefully assessed when deciding on the most appropriate type of support.

Possible Solutions
- Height adjustable armrest
- Padded armrest
- Flat padded armrest
- Molded armrest
- Elevating molded armrest
- Otto Bock armrests (Otto Bock)
- Wheelchair table
    Wooden wheelchair table
    Clear lap tray (Special Health Systems)
- SHS swing-away tray (Special Health Systems)

Height Adjustable Armrest
Height adjustable armrests optimize armrest fit to the individual client. Correctly adjusted armrests provide support to the upper extremities and help the client maintain an upright position.

When using any type of arm trough, adjustable height armrests allow both armrests to remain at the same height.

Armrests that are too low may encourage a kyphotic or scoliotic posture. The client leans forward to rest both upper extremities on the armrests or sideways when resting one upper extremity on one armrest. Armrests that are too high will push upward on the shoulders or clients may keep their upper extremities on their lap encouraging a kyphotic posture. Armrests that are too high will also make mobilizing the wheelchair with the upper extremities difficult.

Height adjustable armrests are an option that is available on most types of wheelchairs. Adjustments usually start from lower than the standard height of 25 cm (10 in.) to much higher. For correct armrest height, see Chapter 2 (Basic Sitting Position in a Wheelchair).

Padded Armrest
The padded armrest is designed to provide good support to the affected upper extremity and especially to the shoulder. It is usually ineffective when there is severe hypertonicity of the upper extremity as the arm tends to be held close to the chest and, consequently, off the armrest.

It may be inappropriate for clients who have severe heminegligence as the limb

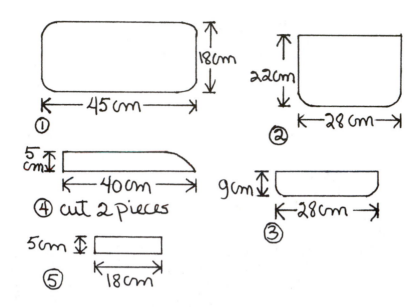

Figure 5-99. Diagram of armrest.

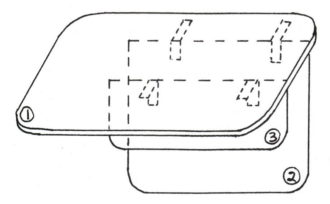

Figure 5-100. Left armrest.

will not be positioned within the visual field.

This type of armrest can be easily fitted to any type of adult wheelchair that has full-length armrests and can be easily removed.

Construction:

1. The padded armrest is made of 1 cm (3/8 in.) plywood.
2. Cut the following pieces as shown in Figure 5-99.
3. Piece 2 is 3 cm (1.25 in.) from the edge of piece 1. Piece 2 is fixed to piece 1 with two corner braces 3 cm (1.25 in.) and screws. Piece 3 is 5.5 cm (2.25 in.) from piece 2. Piece 3 is fixed to piece 1 with two corner braces 3 cm (1.25 in.) and screws (Figure 5-100).

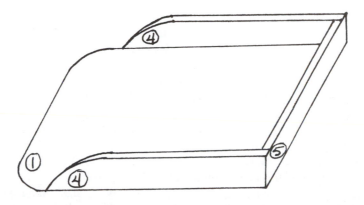

Figure 5-101. Top of the armrest.

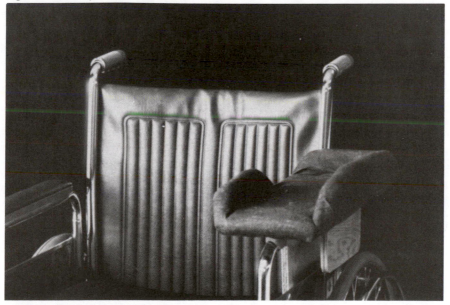

Figure 5-102. Left padded armrest.

4. Pieces 4 and 5 are fixed to piece 1 with glue and screws (Figure 5-101).
5. The armrest is padded with 2.5 cm (1 in.) low density foam. The foam is stapled to the armrest.
6. The padded armrest can be covered with any resistant fabric such as denim. The cover is stapled to the armrest (Figure 5-102).

Flat Padded Armrest

The flat padded armrest provides good support for the weak or flaccid upper extremity especially to the shoulder. It is also recommended in cases of mild hypertonicity of the upper limb.

On this support the arm is held within the immediate visual field. It can be easily fitted to any type of wheelchair with full length armrests and can be easily removed.

Construction:

1. The flat padded armrest is made of 1 cm (3/8 in.) plywood.
2. Cut the following pieces as shown in Figure 5-103.
3. Piece 2 is 3 cm (1.25 in.) from the edge of piece 1. Piece 2 is fixed to piece 1 with two corner braces 3 cm (1.25 in.) and screws. Piece 3 is 5.5 cm (2.25 in.) from piece 2. Piece 2 is fixed to piece 1 with two corner braces 3 cm (1.25 in.) and screws (Figure 5-104).
4. The flat armrest is padded with 2.5 cm (1 in.) low density foam.
5. The flat padded armrest can be covered with any resistant fabric such as denim. The cover is stapled to the armrest (Figure 5-105).

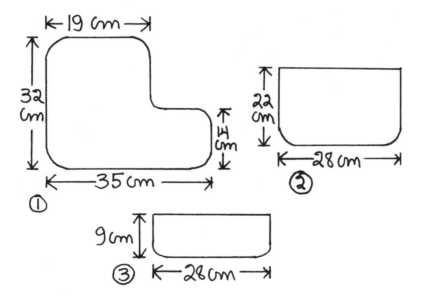

Figure 5-103. Diagram of flat armrest.

Molded Armrest

The molded armrest provides good support to the affected upper extremity, especially to the shoulder.

It is usually ineffective when there is severe hypertonicity of the upper extremity as the arm tends to be held close to the chest, and consequently, off the armrest.

It may be inappropriate for clients with severe heminegligence as the affected extremity will not be held within the visual field.

The molded armrest can be fitted to any type of adult wheelchair with full-length armrests.

Although the molded armrest can be easily removed from the wheelchair, it is usually left in place because it does not interfere with transfers.

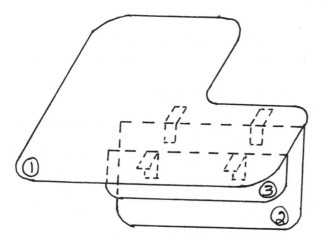

Figure 5-104. Left flat armrest.

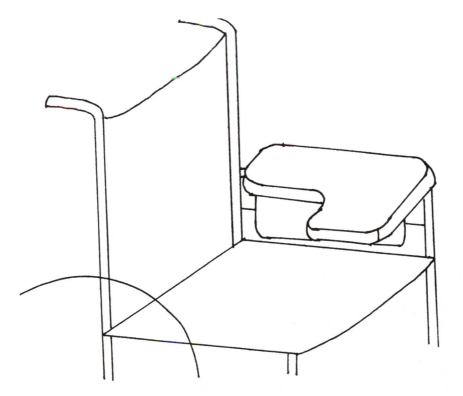

Figure 5-105. Left flat padded armrest.

Construction:

1. The molded armrest is made of a strong, thick, high temperature thermoplastic material such as Uvex 0.3 cm (1/8 in.).
2. Cut the following piece as shown in Figure 5-106. Six slots 5.5 x 0.5 cm (2.25 x 1/5 in.) are cut according to Figure 5-106.
3. Using a wooden block 14 x 7 x 46 cm (5.5 x 2.75 x 18 in.), mold the armrest to bend the two outer sides at 90 degree angles following the dotted lines on Figure 5-106.
4. Make three straps with 5 cm (2 in.) wide webbing, Velcro, and 5 cm (2 in.) long stainless "D" rings. The length of webbing used is 27 cm (10.5 in.). The overall length of the finished strap is 23 cm (9 in.). The three webbing straps (Figure 5-107) fit in the slots of the armrest to fix the armrest to the wheelchair (Figure 5-108).
5. A foam pad of 14 x 46 cm (5.5 x 18 in.) is made of 2.5 cm (1 in.) low density foam. The foam pad is covered with a thin, stretchable fabric such as stockinette. The foam pad is added to the armrest for comfort.

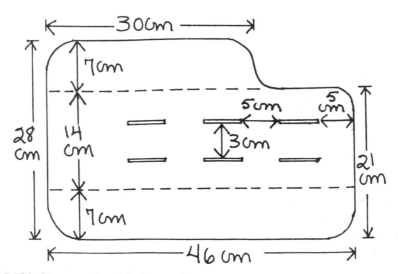

Figure 5-106. Diagram of molded armrest.

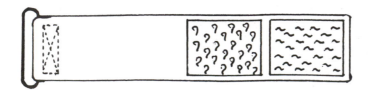

Figure 5-107. Webbing strap.

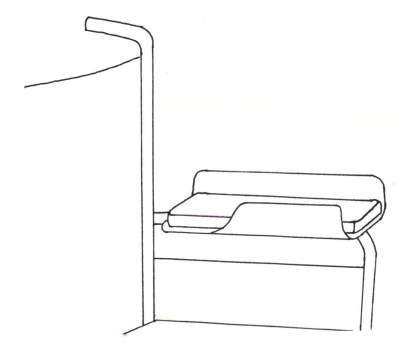

Figure 5-108. Left molded armrest.

Elevating Molded Armrest

The elevating armrest is designed to control edema in the hand. It can be fitted to any type of adult wheelchair that has full-length armrests.

Although the elevating armrest can be easily removed, it is usually left in place because it does not interfere with transfers.

Construction:

1. The elevating armrest is constructed in the same way as the molded armrestwith an added small wooden bridge to provide the elevation. See page 124 (Upper Extremities, Molded Armrest).
2. The wooden bridge is made of 2.5 cm (1 in.) thick wood.
3. Cut the following piece as shown in Figure 5-109.
4. The bridge is fixed to the molded armrest with two screws and rests on the armrest pad of the wheelchair (Figure 5-110). The closer the bridge is placed to the elbow, the greater the elevation of the armrest. The closer the bridge is placed to the hand, the lower the elevation (Figure 5-111).
5. The length of the straps needed to tightly secure the elevating armrest to the wheelchair will need to be increased.

Otto Bock Armrests (Otto Bock)

The Otto Bock armrest can be used for most positioning problems of the upper

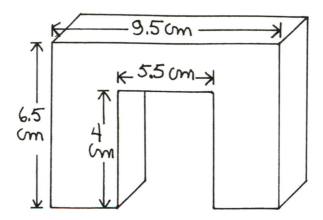

Figure 5-109. Wooden bridge.

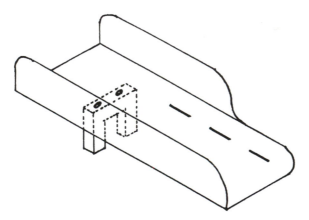

Figure 5-110. Left elevating molded armrest.

extremity. It is easily adjusted to meet individual needs.

Using the elevating swivel unit, the armrest can be inclined 12 or 25 degrees for control of hand edema. Leaving the swivel unit unlocked permits the armrests to swing freely thus accommodating the upper extremity and the client's body movements. This is an advantage for the spastic extremity as it tends to remain on the armrest and for the client with perceptual deficits as the affected extremity will stay within the immediate visual field.

Otto Bock offers a wide selection of armrests. The channel armrest is a one-piece unit which provides support to the forearm but very little for the hand. It is available in one size only. The modular channel armrest features a two-piece arm pad concept (Figure 5-112) that allows three sizes of forearm section to be combined with four different types of hand pad. The forearm pad can be used without the hand pad for

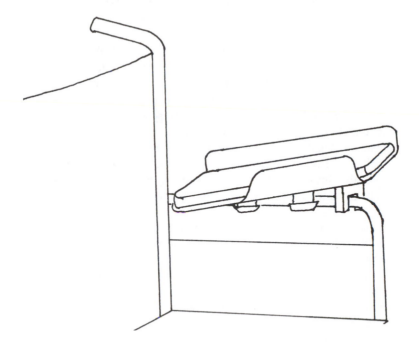

Figure 5-111. Attached elevating molded armrest.

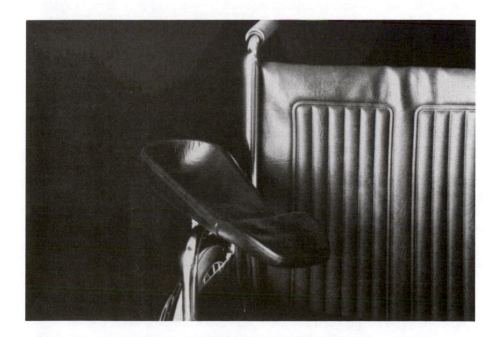

Figure 5-112. Otto Bock modular channel armrest with flat hand pad.

custom mounting or to promote the use of the hand. The four types of hand pad are:
- Flat hand pad: available in medium and large sizes. The flat hand pad is used for the weak or flaccid hand that does not have flexion contractures.
- Palm extensor modular hand pad: available in one size. Specify right or left. It is designed to provide hand support with the fingers in slight flexion. It should not be used if fingers are held in flexion due to hypertonicity or flexion contractures.
- Cone-type modular hand pad: available in one size. Specify right or left. For the upper extremity with mild hypertonicity, it provides positioning for hand and fingers with the forearm held in the mid-position.
- Horn-type modular hand pad: available in one size. Specify right or left. It provides good support for the hypertonic upper extremity by allowing additional fingers and hand support with the forearm pronated. The mounting hardware, the elevating/swivel unit, can be fitted to any type of wheelchair and armrest.

Assembly:

In order to find the appropriate position for the armrest on the wheelchair, the client is first seated in the wheelchair and the armrest pad removed. The Otto Bock is mounted on the wheelchair armrest frame and the swivel unit is unlocked, allowing the armrest to move freely. Then, the upper extremity is placed on the armrest.

The elevating/swivel unit can be moved forward or backward to determine the position that provides the most comfortable support for the upper extremity, especially for the shoulder. To confirm the fit, check the client's sitting posture. The upper trunk must be upright and resting against the back canvas with the shoulders level. The shoulders should be in 30 degrees of flexion with 60 degrees of flexion at the elbow.

When the most appropriate position is found, the elevating/swivel unit is tightly secured to the wheelchair armrest frame. The swivel unit may be locked into one position or left to swing freely.

Wheelchair Table

The wheelchair table can be used for any positioning problem of the upper extremity. It provides good support and permits the affected upper extremity to stay within the immediate visual field. It can also assist the client in maintaining the upright position by providing support and stability to the upper trunk when the forearms and elbows are resting on the table.

A clear plastic wheelchair table will not obstruct the lower extremities from the visual field and will help to maintain body awareness. A wheelchair table facilitates meal management and table activities but will interfere with the ability to transfer independently. It may also restrict independent wheelchair mobility with the non-affected upper extremity if the wheelchair table extends beyond the armrests.

Wheelchair tables can be fitted to any type of adult wheelchair with full-length armrests.

Wooden Wheelchair Table
Construction:
1. Use 0.5 cm (1/4 in.) plywood and 1 x 1.5 cm (0.5 x 0.75 in.) wooden strips.
2. To fit a 41 cm (16 in.) wide adult wheelchair or a 46 cm (18 in.) wide wheelchair,

cut the following pieces as shown in Figure 5-113. On piece 1, make two slots of 1 x 5 cm (0.5 x 2 in.) according to Figure 5-113.

3. Pieces 2 and 3 are glued and nailed to piece 1 according to Figure 5-114.

4. Make two straps with 5 cm (2 in.) wide Velcro. The strap is made of one piece 30 cm (12 in.) long loop and 7.5 cm (3 in.) long hook. The straps are stapled to the wheelchair table according to Figure 5-114.

5. The wooden wheelchair table (Figure 5-115) should be sanded and varnished for a good finish and for ease of cleaning.

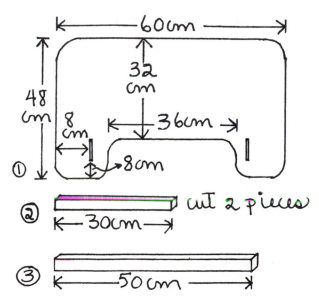

Figure 5-113. Diagram of wooden wheelchair table.

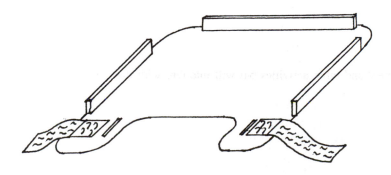

Figure 5-114. Wooden wheelchair table.

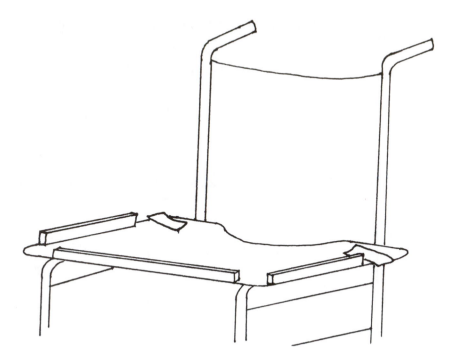

Figure 5-115. Wooden wheelchair table.

Clear Lap Tray (Special Health Systems)
Assembly:
The SHS clear lap tray is available in one standard size to fit any adult wheelchair 41 and 46 cm (16 and 18 in.) wide with full-length armrests. It is attached to the wheelchair armrests with two Velcro straps.

The clear lap tray (Figure 5-116) has a removable rubber trim to encourage awareness of the edge of the tray.

The clear lap tray has the advantage of permitting the client to see the lower extremities thus providing greater body awareness.

SHS Swing-Away Tray (Special Health Systems)
The SHS swing-away tray (Figure 5-117) is designed to provide support to one affected upper extremity and to its shoulder. It permits the affected upper extremity to stay within the immediate visual field. The clear plastic tray will not obstruct the lower extremities from the visual field and will help to maintain body awareness. It has a white rubber trim to encourage awareness of the edge of the tray.

The swing-away tray is less than half the size of the SHS clear lap tray (Special Health Systems). The swing-away tray is available in one standard size to fit any adult wheelchair with full-length armrests. It is necessary to specify right or left armrest. With the armrest pad removed, it attaches to the armrest with a bracket. The

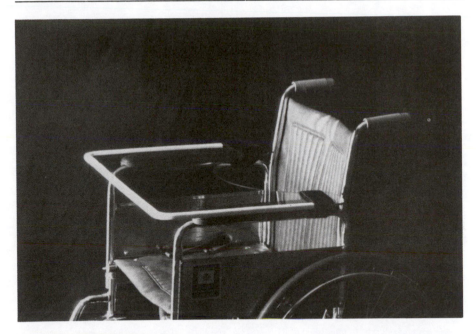

Figure 5-116. Clear lap tray.

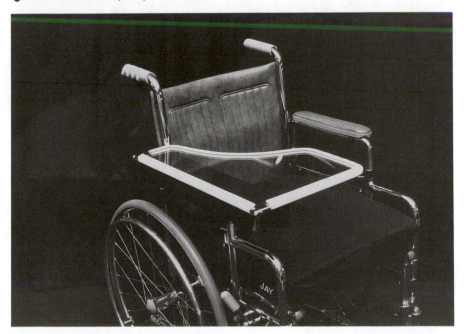

Figure 5-117. Right SHS swing-away tray.

swing-away tray easily swings around over the wheelchair wheel to allow for independent standing transfers.

6 Custom Molded Seating Insert

The following is intended to be an open discussion on custom molded seating inserts to assist the therapist when deciding whether or not to prescribe such a seating system. It includes a broad definition of a custom molded seating insert, points to consider, the role of the prescribing therapist, and for whom they are intended.

Custom molded seating inserts are usually prescribed for severely physically disabled clients. These disabilities are often fixed skeletal deformities which can be accompanied by soft tissue contracture and chronic pressure sore problems especially over bony prominences and high abnormal motor activity. Generally, regular types of seating and off-the-shelf seating equipment have failed to meet the client's positioning and seating needs.

Custom molded seating inserts are designed to provide an anatomically contoured seat, which maximizes contact with the body; to distribute the weight over the greatest possible surface; to provide support; and to optimize correction. The seating insert is usually mounted on a wheelchair or any type of wheeled chassis. The rigid structure of the seating insert prevents movement between the body and the seat which would result in the contour of the seat not matching the client's body.

Several approaches and methods have been devised to fabricate custom molded seating inserts and different types of material are used. The two main methods are:
- Direct molding of the insert on the client.
- Making a plaster mold of the client using a rubber bag, such as a weather balloon, filled with polystyrene beads and an air compressor. The plaster mold is then used to fabricate a seating insert made of molded foam or other type of material such as the Matrix system.

Direct Molding

Seating inserts can be made using the expansion of a two-part, semi-rigid polyurethane foam within an elastic envelope. Another type of insert uses a rubber bag, such as a weather balloon, containing polystyrene beads. The seat is molded by adding a slow curing flexible epoxy resin to the beads and an air compressor to hold the shape of the mold until the epoxy has cured.[7] The insert can be molded while placed directly into the wheelchair, or it can be mounted on an interface that can be made of wood or strong ABS thermoplastic material and fixed to the chair using webbing straps or aluminum tubing and clamps. The molding time will vary according to the setting time of the material used. It can range from 20 minutes to approximately an hour and a half. The molding time is the time available to hand mold the bag into an approximate supportive shape plus the time when the client then sits on the newly molded seat bag to attain maximum conformity, support, and comfort. Once the material has set, the bag can be peeled away and minor modifications can be made using a knife.

Plaster Molding/Vacuum Consolidation

Seating inserts can be made from a plaster mold of the client. One method of taking a plaster mold is to use a rubber bag, such as a weather balloon, filled with polystyrene beads and an air compressor. The rubber bag is usually placed in the client's wheelchair. Some air is removed from the bag using the air compressor until the bag can be worked into the predetermined shape of the client but without being completely solid. The client is then seated on the rubber bag. When the molding and shaping of the seat is completed, all air is removed from the bag using the air compressor until the seat is fully rigid and maintains the molded shape. The client is then transferred out of the new seat. A plaster mold is taken from the shaped rubber bag using plaster bandages. From the positive plaster mold, a seating insert can be made from material such as the expansion of a two-part, semi-rigid polyurethane foam or the Matrix body support system.

Advantages and Disadvantages

- Absence of flexibility for adjustment and modifications to adapt to changes in the client's status. A seating insert has a fixed shape. Only minor modifications can be done compared to off-the-shelf seating equipments which can be fitted and adjusted in any environment without a workshop facility.
- When off-the-shelf seating equipment fails to meet the seating needs of a severely disabled client, a custom molded seating insert will often provide better support and comfort.
- To make custom molded seating inserts, skill and experience are required. Asking for assistance from a specialized seating clinic is strongly advised. The cost of

material added to the specialized service makes a seating insert relatively expensive. However, a well-customized system can last several years, in which case the expense is justifiable.

- The technique of direct molding a seating insert has the advantage of limiting the amount of material needed to make the insert. As well, it is a faster process with less steps than using the vacuum consolidation casting technique. Cost of direct molding can be kept to a minimum in material and specialist time. The main disadvantage of direct molding resides in the fact that the time for molding and shaping the final seat is limited and does not allow for trial and error.

- The vacuum consolidation casting technique requires more material, time, and steps than the technique of direct molding and, therefore, is usually more expensive. The main advantage is that the molding time is limited only by the client's ability to tolerate the procedure which can be spread over a few sessions. The rubber bag and air compressor can be used to determine if a custom molded seating insert is an appropriate solution to meet the seating needs of an individual client.

Steps to Making a Custom Molded Seating Insert

Assessment

The primary therapists, i.e., occupational therapist and physiotherapist, gather all information relevant to the decision-making process. If a custom molded seating insert is chosen, then goals and objectives are established. This process must be client centered and involve the primary caregiver(s).

The assessment includes:

- Diagnosis and prognosis.
- Client's present level of functioning. Ability to transfer in and out of the wheelchair, wheelchair mobility, activities of daily living, occupation, interests and hobbies.
- Continence.
- Skin integrity, pressure sores, history of pressure sores. Note location(s).
- Physical assessment. Include passive and active range of motion, contractures, deformity, tone, strength, pain.
- An assessment of the client's sitting position. What is the optimal sitting position that is comfortable and promotes function? The sitting position must be as symmetric as possible to promote even loading on both sides of the body, to maintain alignment of the spine, head and neck and to bring the upper extremities into a midline position. How much upright sitting is possible? What is the present sitting tolerance?
- The present and possible future need for specialized equipment such as communication and environmental control devices, computer.
- What has been tried in terms of positioning, wheelchairs, and equipment? Why was it unsatisfactory or unsuccessful?

- Environment. Where is the seating system going to be used? Indoors versus outdoors? Small space, such as an apartment, versus large space, such as an institution?
- Transportation. Does the seating system need to be dismantled for ease of transport?

Establish Goals and Objectives

In terms of seating and posture, what can be achieved? For example, a goal might be to control high extensor tone, providing trunk and head support. Features can be molded into the seating insert to meet specific needs of the client.

What abilities are to be maintained or promoted in the areas of activities of daily living, communication, mobility, occupation, and leisure?

Molding

In collaboration with a molded seating insert specialist, a decision is made regarding which method to use, i.e., direct molding or vacuum consolidation casting technique, as well as the type of material to be used to fabricate the seating insert. The decision is based on the specialist's knowledge of the advantages and disadvantages of various materials and techniques combined with the therapist's assessment of the client.

An initial molding is done. As much as possible, this is completed in an environment familiar to the client to avoid undue stress, fatigue, and excitement involved with traveling to a seating clinic and a new environment. The client may need a rest period if the molding requires a long time.

Workshop Fabrication

This includes the fabrication of the molded seating insert, cover(s), fitting the insert to a wheelchair or wheeled chassis, and the possible addition of lap belt, tray, or other accessories.

Final Fitting

This step is to confirm the fit of the newly fabricated custom molded seating insert. When the system is received, the following should be checked:

- Condition of the seating system. Structural breakdown of support and damage to the seat surface.
- Adjustment and functioning of accessories.
- When appropriate, how the chair is dismantled.

The client should be transferred to the seating system and the following checked:

- How the client transfers in and out of the chair and if there is any difficulty in moving.
- That the seat holds the client in a functional position.
- That the seat is comfortable: temperature, softness of seating surface. What is the initial reaction of the client? How does the client first adjust? Does the client feel satisfied with the new seat?
- After spending approximately 30 minutes in the new seat, the client is checked for

redness of the skin indicating pressure area(s).

Finally, the therapist provides demonstration and information to the primary caregiver(s) on how to use the new custom molded seating system and accessories. Goals and objectives are reviewed and a follow-up seating plan is decided upon for the period when the client is adapting and adjusting to the seating system.

Follow Up

Refer to Chapter 7 for indications on how to proceed and suggested time frame. The therapist also checks the following:

- Condition of the seating system and accessories. Are changes necessary? Adjustments? Only minor changes can be made to the structure and the insert. Contact the specialist responsible for the fabrication to carry out any changes and modifications.
- Check the seat for comfort: temperature, softness of the seating surface, contour and fit, skin redness.
- Does the seat still provide the client with a functional sitting position? Are there any changes in the client's level of functioning? What are they? Can the seating system and accessories be modified to better meet the needs of the client?
- Are the client and primary caregiver(s) still satisfied with the seating system?
- Lastly, review the goals and objectives, and the initial follow-up seating plan. Modify accordingly and as needed in collaboration with the client and primary caregiver(s).

For severely disabled clients who have complex positioning problems a custom molded seating insert may be the best viable option. It is possible that new areas of function which were latent or underdeveloped may become apparent. Custom molded seating inserts are not meant for everybody as they provide only one unique sitting position which does not allow for movement in the chair or easy modification. Clients must be precisely positioned in the system to maximize support and comfort, and therefore, caregivers require special instructions. Custom inserts should be used only when ready-made seating equipment have failed to meet the needs of the individual client.

7 Follow Up

Without follow up, positioning may fail. Clients take time to adjust to a new sitting position. The length of time will vary according to the situation. A slight adjustment to a new adaptation can make the difference between success and failure.

A new technique or device should be tried in the morning and early in the week to allow for good follow up. If the client is positioned on a Friday and left for the weekend without monitoring, potential problems could arise. This could result in the complete rejection of a positioning device and loss of trust. Since new positioning may require a compromise, the client and caregiver might require reassurance.

Step by Step Positioning

For many clients with moderate seating problems, positioning cannot be completed in one session. Finding the most appropriate intervention may be an ongoing process. It may take a few days to a week or longer. In order not to unnecessarily restrict a client's movements, systematically going through a step by step process and getting to the root of the problem may provide a simpler solution. Keeping in mind that the least amount of intervention is preferable, the intention is to facilitate the body's natural ability to maintain the upright position.

For example, a client is referred with the problem of constantly sliding down in the wheelchair and leaning to the side. On assessment, shortening of the hamstrings is identified with the resulting limitation of hip flexion and knee extension. To accommodate the short hamstrings, the client slides down in the wheelchair to increase knee flexion. Is the leaning a result of that same process? The presenting problem may not be where you need to start to work.

- The first step is to provide a base of support. The pelvis and thighs are positioned with an appropriate cushion. To avoid stretching the hamstrings thus allowing increased hip flexion and decreased the tone, no foot support is provided.
- Foot support is provided where the feet fall.
- When the lower body is well positioned and stable, the client is reassessed for sliding and leaning. Is a safety belt still required? Lateral support?

Instead of providing a safety belt and a lateral support at the beginning and thus limiting trunk mobility, using the step by step method has helped to determine that providing an appropriate base for the pelvis and then foot support where it is needed to accommodate the short hamstrings may be all that is required. Unless the root of the problem is discovered, unnecessary adaptations could be used to solve the presenting problem(s) but will not address the underlying cause(s).

When many caregivers are involved with a client, labeling a device clearly to indicate the way it should be positioned on the wheelchair is vital to its successful use. Diagrams and instructions at the bedside help new staff or casual relief staff to use the device appropriately.

Depending on the system in use, charting is essential. A communication book, cardex, and charting are good methods to communicate problems and plans. Keeping a record of solutions that have been tried may expedite the work of other therapists at a future date.

Once a satisfactory position is determined check the client:

- The first day—at noon and in the late afternoon.
- The first week—twice a day, once in the morning to make sure the device is applied correctly and after a few hours to observe the effects of fatigue.
- Once a week for the first month.
- Every 6 months or whenever there is a major change in the client physical status. This also provides the therapist with the opportunity to check that all devices and equipment are in good condition and still being used properly.

Regularly scheduled in-services on the importance of positioning are critical. Unless the primary caregivers understand why a certain device is necessary it will be little used. Once the benefits to the client and caregivers are understood compliance may not be a problem and feedback on the success of the intervention will be assured.

Good follow up is an integral part of the positioning process and will ensure success.

8 Conclusion

Adaptive seating should be considered an extension of the individual treatment program and as such should support the goals of the treatment plan. Technology is changing constantly and new devices are on the market every month. Careful assessment of the needs of the client combined with the knowledge of available adaptive equipment will lead to good positioning solutions. Local dealers who specialize in medical equipment are often helpful in locating appropriate devices. The therapist who understands the problem will be able to assess the new equipment to determine if it will meet the needs of the client and to identify potential disadvantages.

Because each client is unique, there are no predetermined solutions for specific diagnosis or categories. Positioning, therefore, requires time and patience. Several ideas may be tried before the most appropriate solution is found. The knowledge and skills of each team member combined with good communication create that necessary shared vision. The importance of seating intervention in care facilities has to be recognized because almost all aspects of the client's waking life are affected by positioning in a wheelchair. If we choose to see possibilities and opportunities instead of problems and limitations, it is entirely possible to help the client reconnect with their aliveness.

"Now am I seated as my soul delights..."
William Shakespeare, *Henry VI*

Appendix

List of Manufacturers and Distributors

The following is a list of the manufacturers and distributors for the wheelchairs, seating systems, and adaptations included in this manual.

When ordering a seating system or a wheelchair adaptation it should be verified that the device is compatible with the wheelchair being used. If an adaptation is required for a special type or size of wheelchair it is often possible to have items custom made by the manufacturer.

Everest and Jennings Canadian Ltd.
111 Snidercroft Road
Toronto, Ontario
L4K 1B6 Canada

Everest and Jennings International Ltd.
1100 Corporate Square
St. Louis, Missouri 63132
United States

IDC Tectonics Ltd.
P.O. Box 2104
Station B
St. Catherines, Ontario
L2M 6P5 Canada

Invacare Canada
5970 Chedworth Way
Mississauga, Ontario
L5R 3T9 Canada

Invacare Corp.
899 Cleveland Street
Elyria, Ohio 44036
United States

Jay Medical Ltd.
4745 Walnut
Boulder, Colorado 80301-2537
United States

J.T. Posey Co. Inc.
5635 Peck Road
Arcadia, California 91006
United States

Maddak Inc.
6 Industrial Road
Pequannock, New Jersey 07440
United States

Otto Bock Orthopedic Industry
3000 Xenium Lane North
Minneapolis, Minnesota 55441
United States

Otto Bock Orthopedic Industry of Canada Ltd.
251 Saulteaux Crescent
Winnipeg, Manitoba
R3J 3C7 Canada

QA2 Seating System
Distributor: Anamed Medical Supply Medical Gas
118 South East Marine Drive
Vancouver, British Columbia
V5X 2S3 Canada

Roho Inc.
100 Florida Avenue
Belleville, Illinois 62221
United States

Special Health Systems
90 Englehard Drive
Aurora, Ontario
L4G 3V2 Canada

References

1. Bar, C., Locke, C. & Salmon, P. (1987). Rockwood bead seat. *Physiotherapy, 73*(12), 650-652.
2. Johnson Taylor, S. (1987). Evaluating the client with physical disabilities for wheelchair seating. *American Journal of Occupational Therapy, 41*(11), 711-716.
3. Lewis, J. (Summer 1975). How to select the right wheelchair for you. *Accent on Living*, 64-70.
4. Lipton Garber, S. (1979). A classification of wheelchair seating. *American Journal of Occupational Therapy, 33*(10), 652-654.
5. Lipton Garber, S. (1985). Wheelchair cushions: A historical review. *American Journal of Occupational Therapy, 39*(7), 453-459.
6. Lipton Garber, S., Krouskop, T. A. & Carter, R. E. (1978). A system for clinically evaluating wheelchair pressure-relief cushions. *American Journal of Occupational Therapy, 32*(9), 565-570.
7. Moore, S., et al. (1982). The DESEMO customized seating support-custom molded seating for severely disabled persons. *Physical Therapy, 62*(4), 460-463.

Bibliography

Bardsley, G. I. (1984). The Dundee seating programme. *Physiotherapy, 70*(2), 59-63.

Beck, M. A. & Klayman Callahan, D. (1980). Impact of institutionalization on the posture of chronic schizophrenic patients. *American Journal of Occupational Therapy, 34*(5), 332-335.

Borello-France, D. F., et al. (1988). Modification of sitting posture of patients with hemiplegia using seat boards and back boards. *Physical Therapy, 68*(1), 67-71.

Bradey, E., et al. (1986). A validity study of guidelines for wheelchair selection. *Canadian Journal of Occupational Therapy, 53*(1), 19-24.

Braile, L. E. (1981). Support for the dropping head. *American Journal of Occupational Therapy, 35*(10), 661-662.

Brunswic, M. (1984). Ergonomics of seat design. *Physiotherapy, 70*(2), 40-43.

Crewe, R. A. (1979). Wheelchair choice. *British Journal of Occupational Therapy, 42*(11), 272-274.

Everest and Jennings Inc. (1979). Measuring the patient. *Wheelchair Prescriptions.*

Fourth International Seating Symposium Syllabus. (1988). *Challenges '88—Seating the Disabled.* Sunny Hill Hospital, University of British Columbia, University of Tennessee.

G. F. Strong Rehabilitation Centre. (1980). *Wheelchair Handbook.* Canada: Author.

Gilewich, G. & Paterson, J. S. (1975). Hemiplegic armrest. *Canadian Journal of Occupational Therapy, 42*(2), 63-65.

Gillot, H., et al. (1983). Current thinking on pressure sores. *British Journal of Occupational Therapy, 46*(2), 41-43.

Harms, M. (1990). Effect of wheelchair design on posture and comfort of users. *Physiotherapy, 76*(5), 266-270.

Hilbers, P. A. & White, T. P. (1990). Effects of wheelchair design on metabolic heart rate responses during propulsion by persons with paraplegia. *Physical Therapy,* *76*(3), 187-191.

Hundertmark Hollett, L. (1985). Evaluating the adult with cerebral palsy for specialized adaptive seating. *Physical Therapy, 65*(2), 209-212.

Kamenetz, H. (1969). *The wheelchair book—Mobility for the disabled.* Springfield, IL: Charles C. Thomas.

Karlander, D. (1983). The new generation of wheelchairs. *Physiotherapy, 69*(12), 428-429.

Lewis, J. (November/December 1975). Five tips for successful wheelchair fitting. *Patient Aid Digest,* 18-20.

Majeske, C. & Buchanan, C. (1984). Quantitative description of two sitting postures with and without a lumbar support pillow. *Physical Therapy, 64*(10), 1531-1533.

Mulcahy, C. M., et al. (1988). Adaptive seating for the motor handicapped problems. A solution, assessment and prescription. *Physiotherapy, 74*(10), 531-536.

Nelham, R. L. (1984). Principles and practice in the manufacture of seating for the handicapped. *Physiotherapy, 70*(2), 59-63.

O'Brien, M. & Tsurumi, K. (1983). The effect of two body positions on head righting in severely disabled individuals with cerebral palsy. *American Journal of Occupational Therapy, 37*(10), 673-680.

Otto Bock Orthopedic Industry of Canada Ltd. (1987). *Please, be seated! Current trends for the disabled* (2nd ed.). Canada: Author.

Pope, P. M. (1985). A study of instability in relation to posture in the wheelchair. *Physiotherapy, 71*(3), 124-129.

Pope, P. M. (1985). Proposals for the improvement of the unstable postural condition and some cautionary notes. *Physiotherapy, 71*(3), 129-131.

Settle, C. (1987). Seating and pressures sores. *Physiotherapy, 73*(9), 455-457.

Sharman, A. & Ponton, T. (1990). The social, functional and physiological benefits of intimately-contoured customized seating: The Matrix body support system. *Physiotherapy, 76*(3), 187-191.

Shields, R. K. & Cook, T. M. (1988). Effect of seat angle and lumbar support on seated buttock pressure. *Physical Therapy, 68*(11), 1682-1686.

Steed, A. (1986). Using the Steed cushion in the treatment of flaccid hemiplegia. *British Journal of Occupational Therapy, 49*(2), 34-38.

Warren, G. C., et al. (1982). Reducing back displacement in the powered reclining wheelchair. *Archives of Physical Medicine and Rehabilitation, 63*(9), 447-449.